I0756904

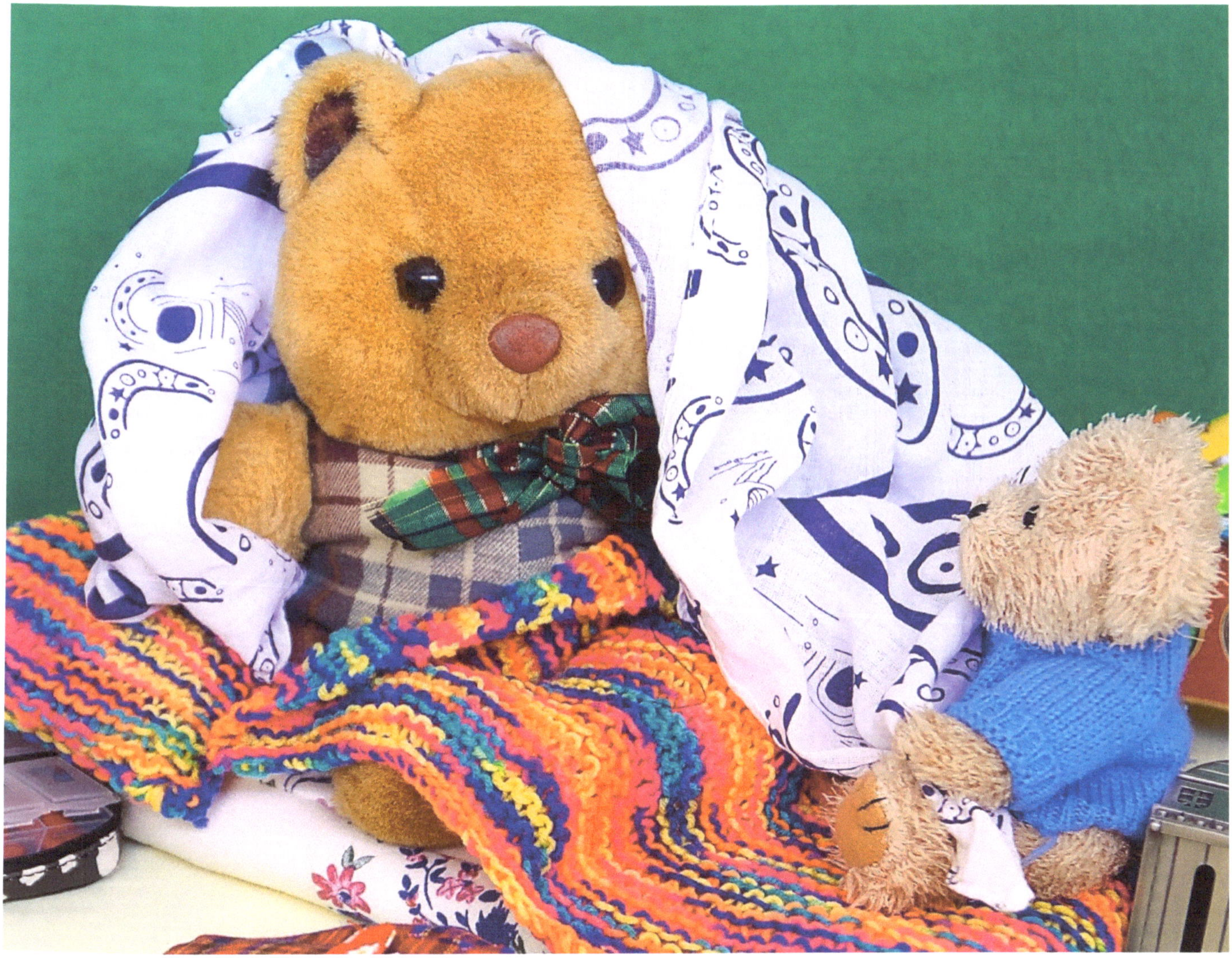

Written by Carola Schmidt

Photographed by Mark O'Dwyer

Edited by Chris Roy

When a Brave Bear Fights Cancer

A GET WELL SOON GIFT

5

What do you do when you feel overwhelmed with doubts and bad news?

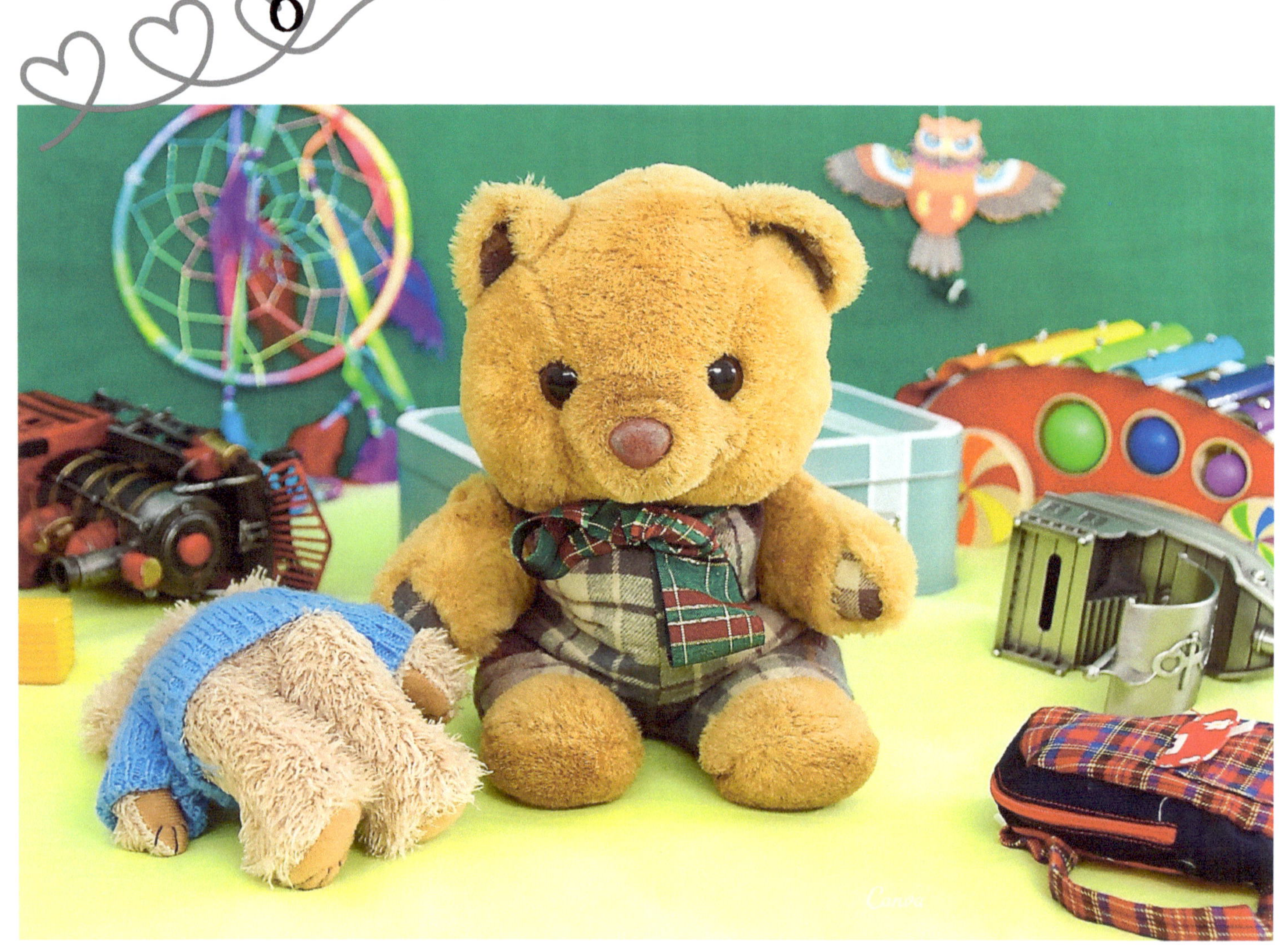

Hold a friend's paw...

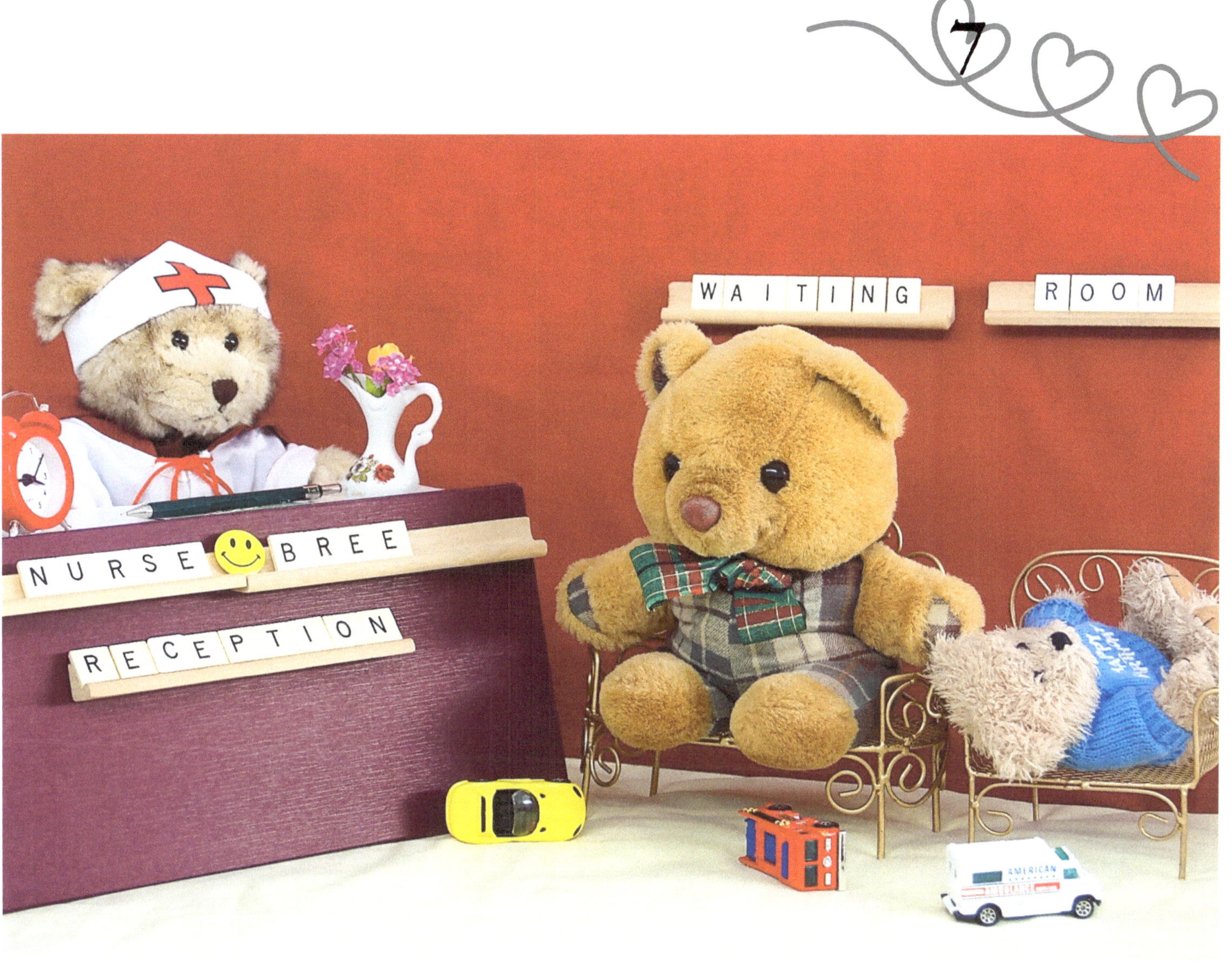

And make your way straight to the cure.

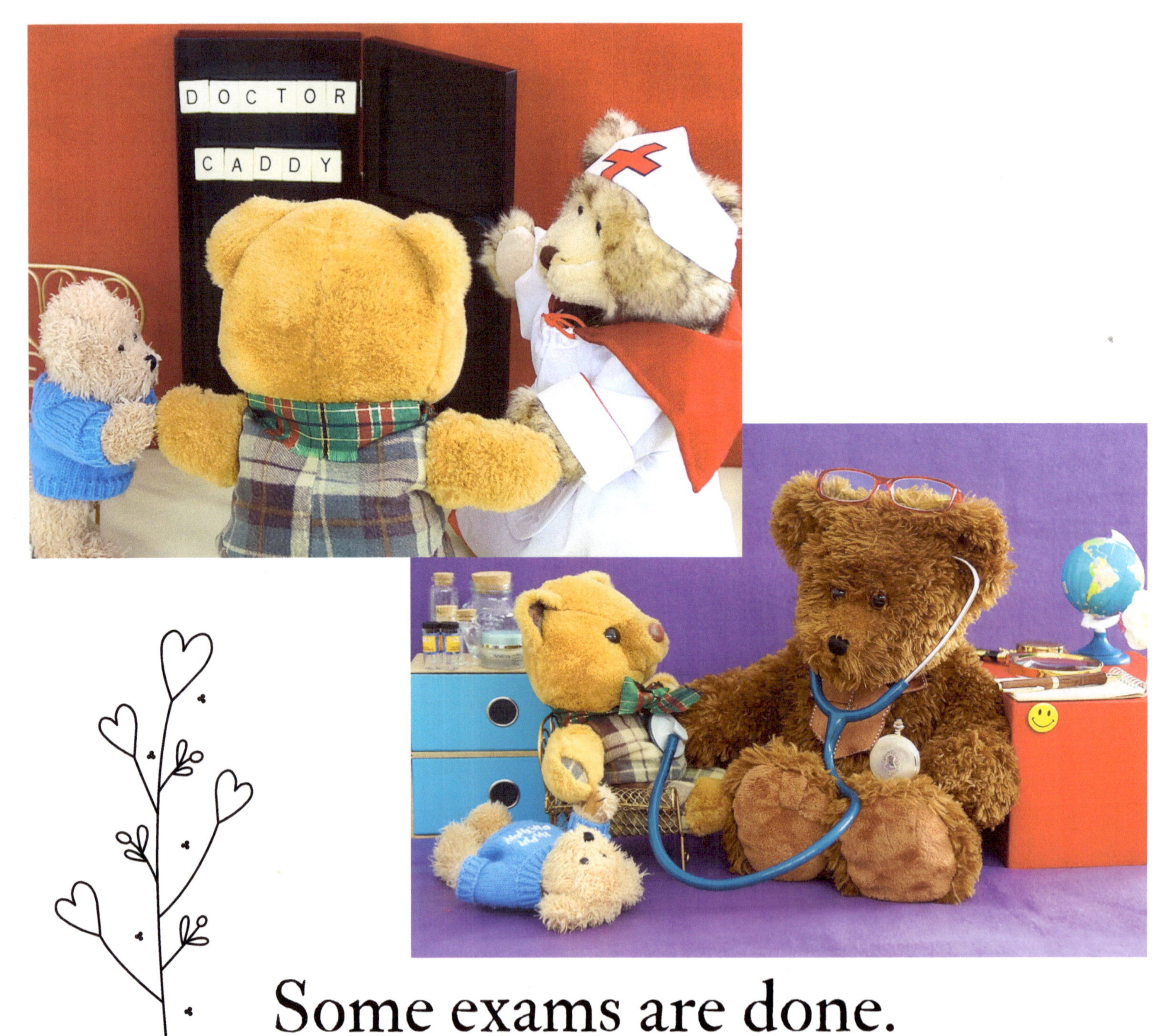

Some exams are done.
Some words are said.

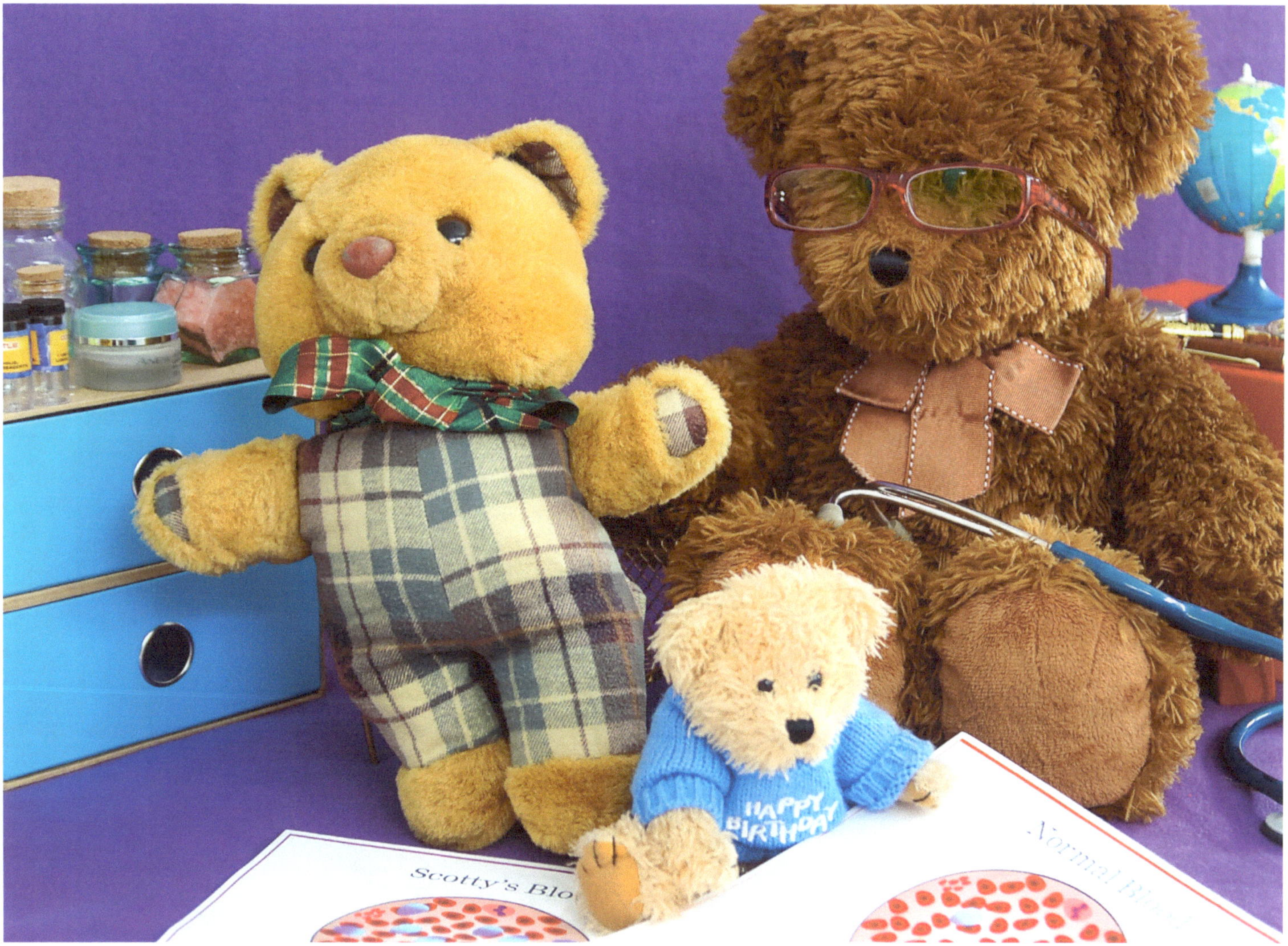

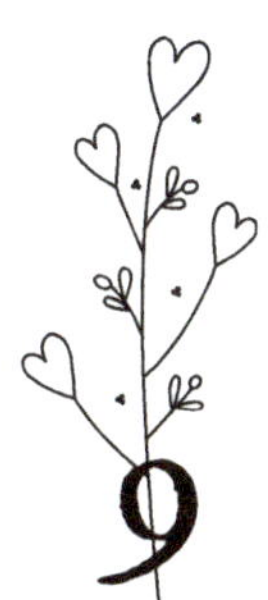

And when you think you might
fall...

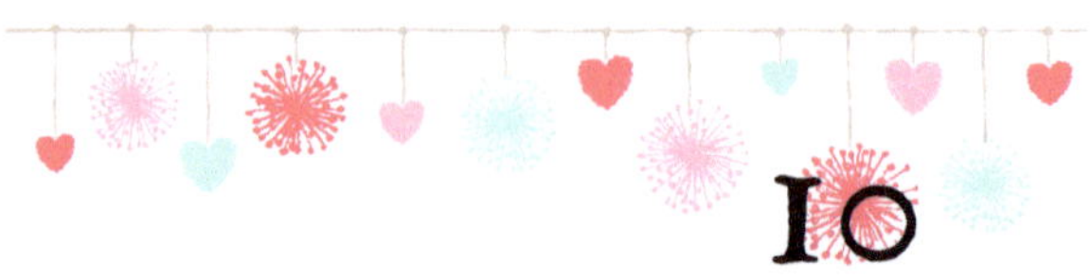

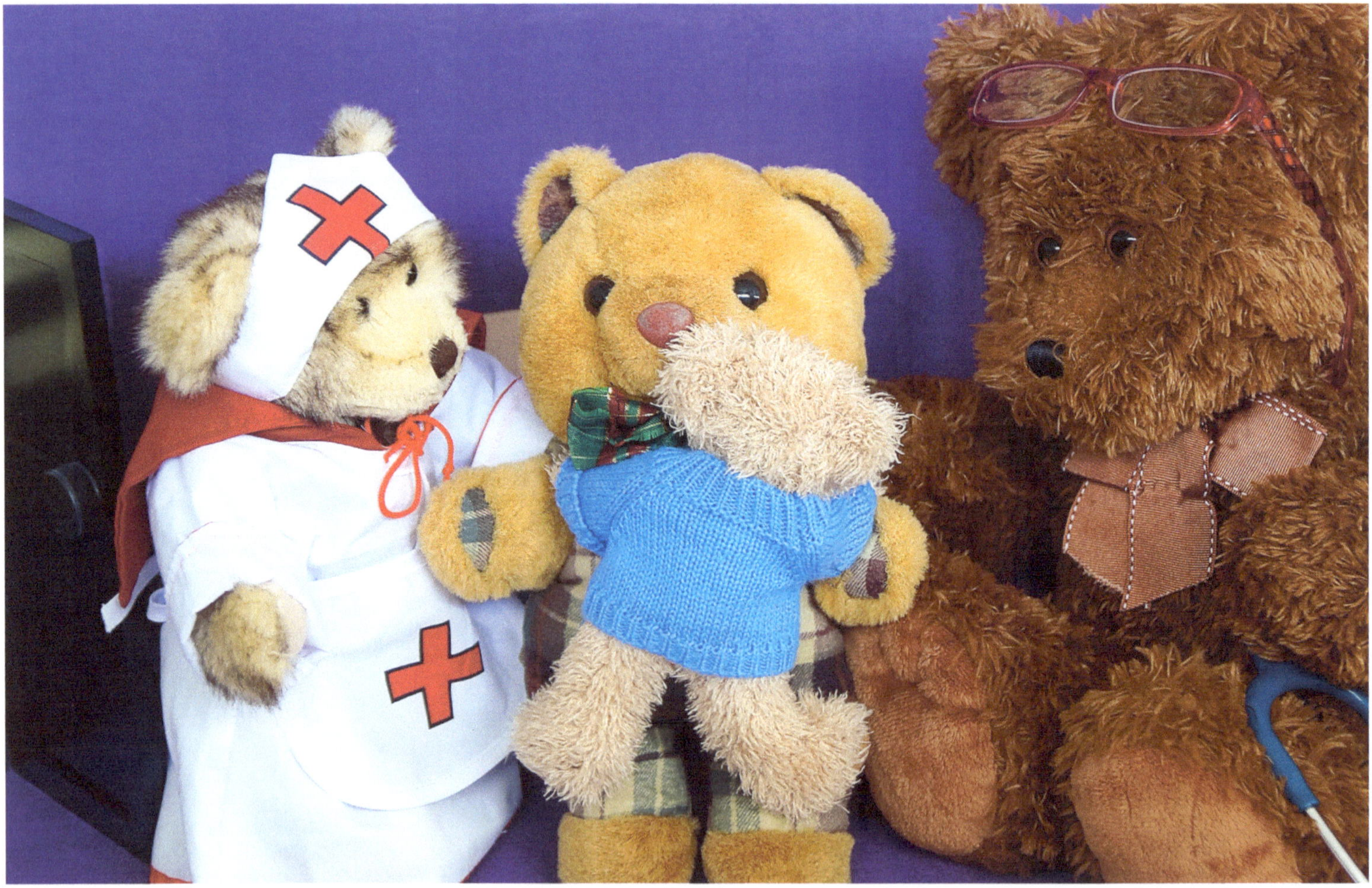

Bear Hugs come your way!

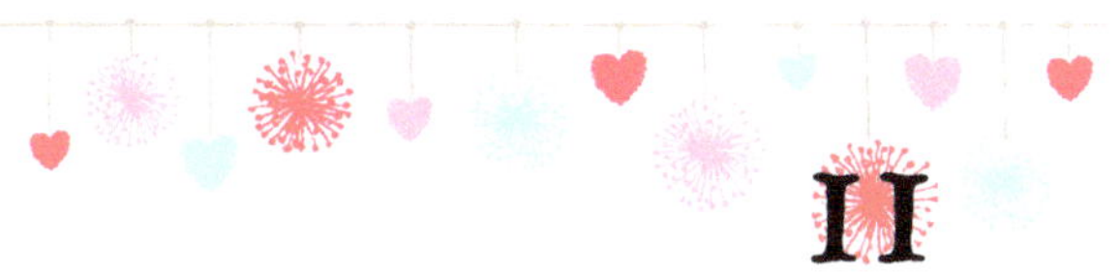

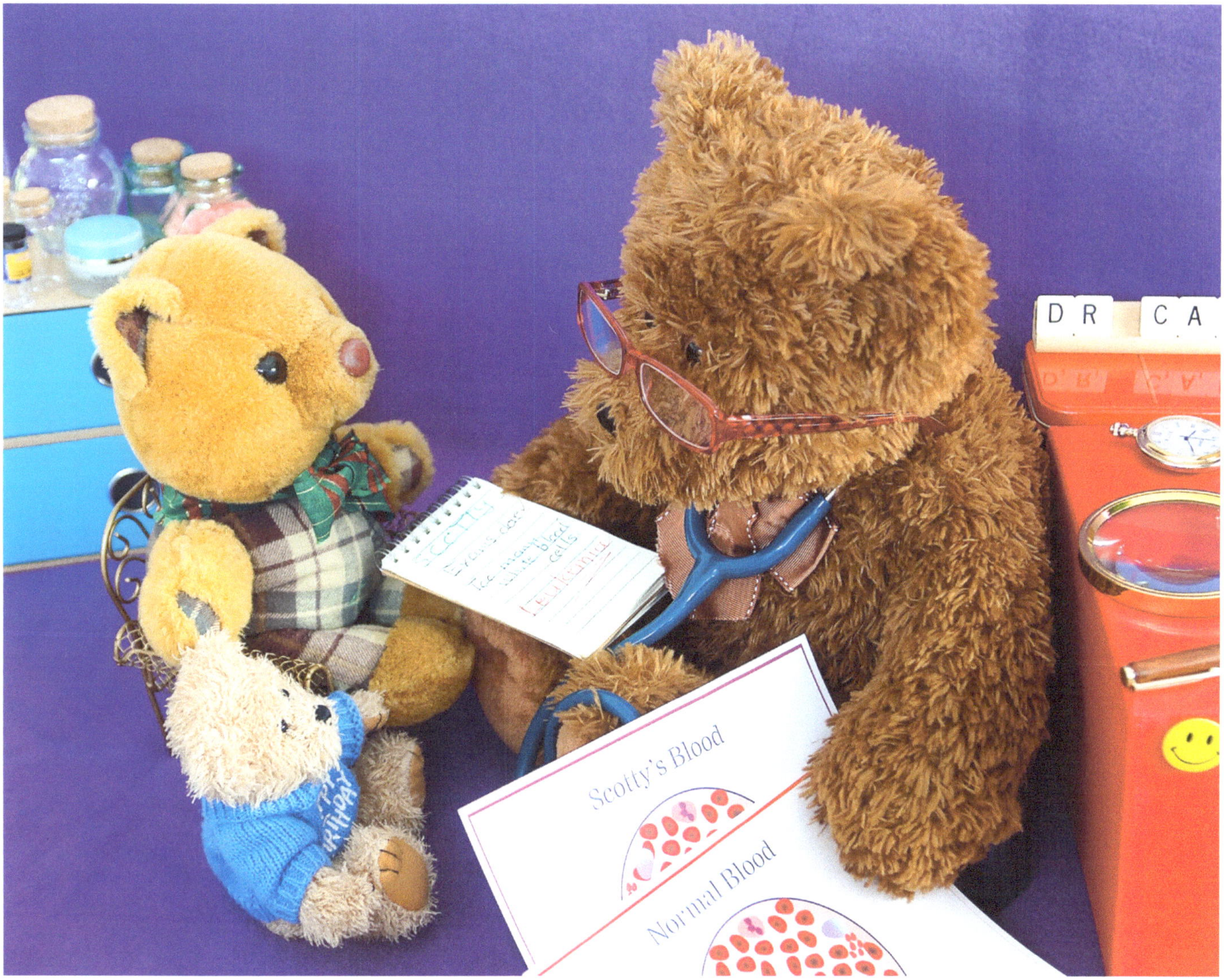

11

The doctor explains the diagnosis,

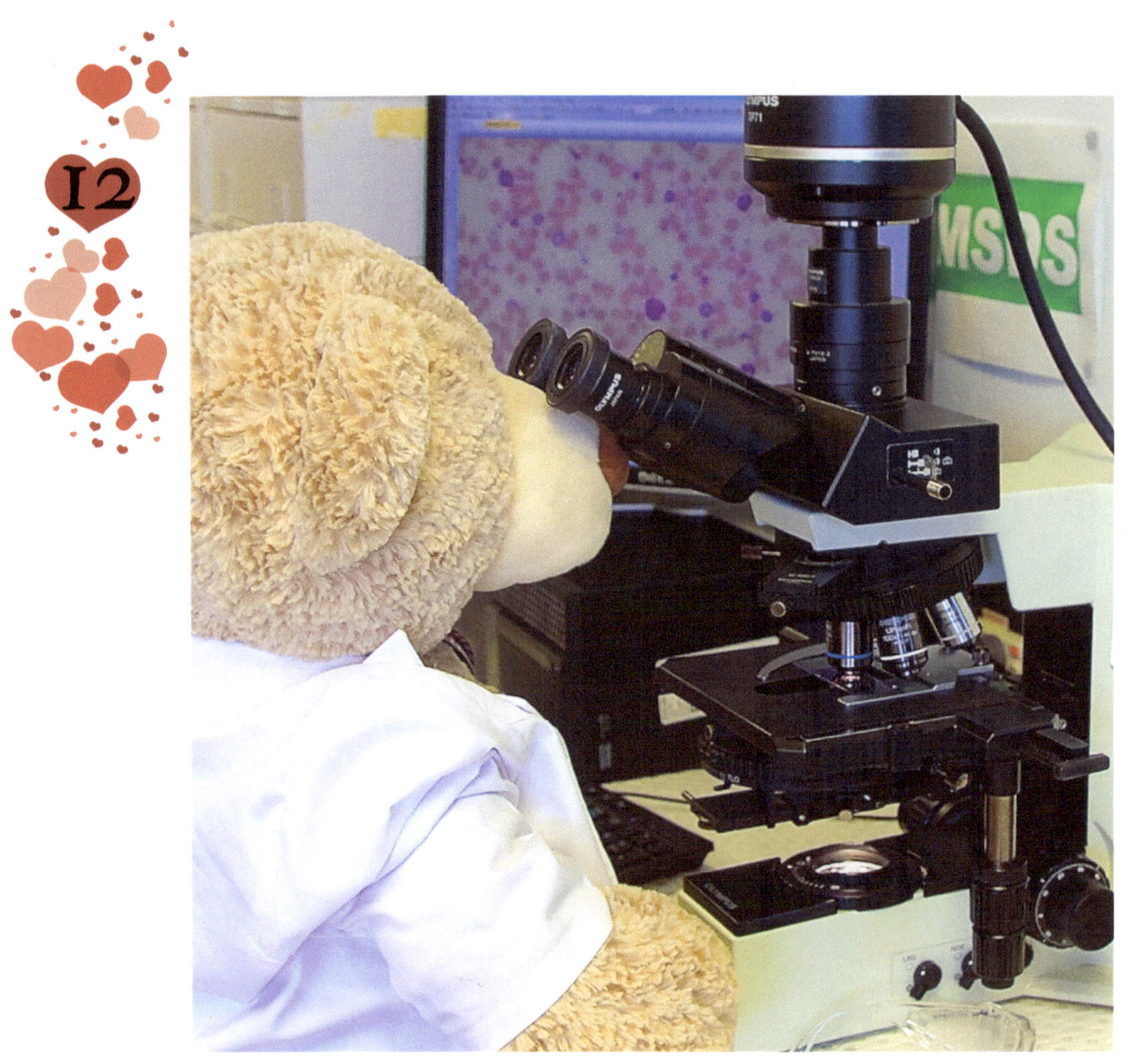

"Your whole body is made of tiny cells. You can see them through a microscope."

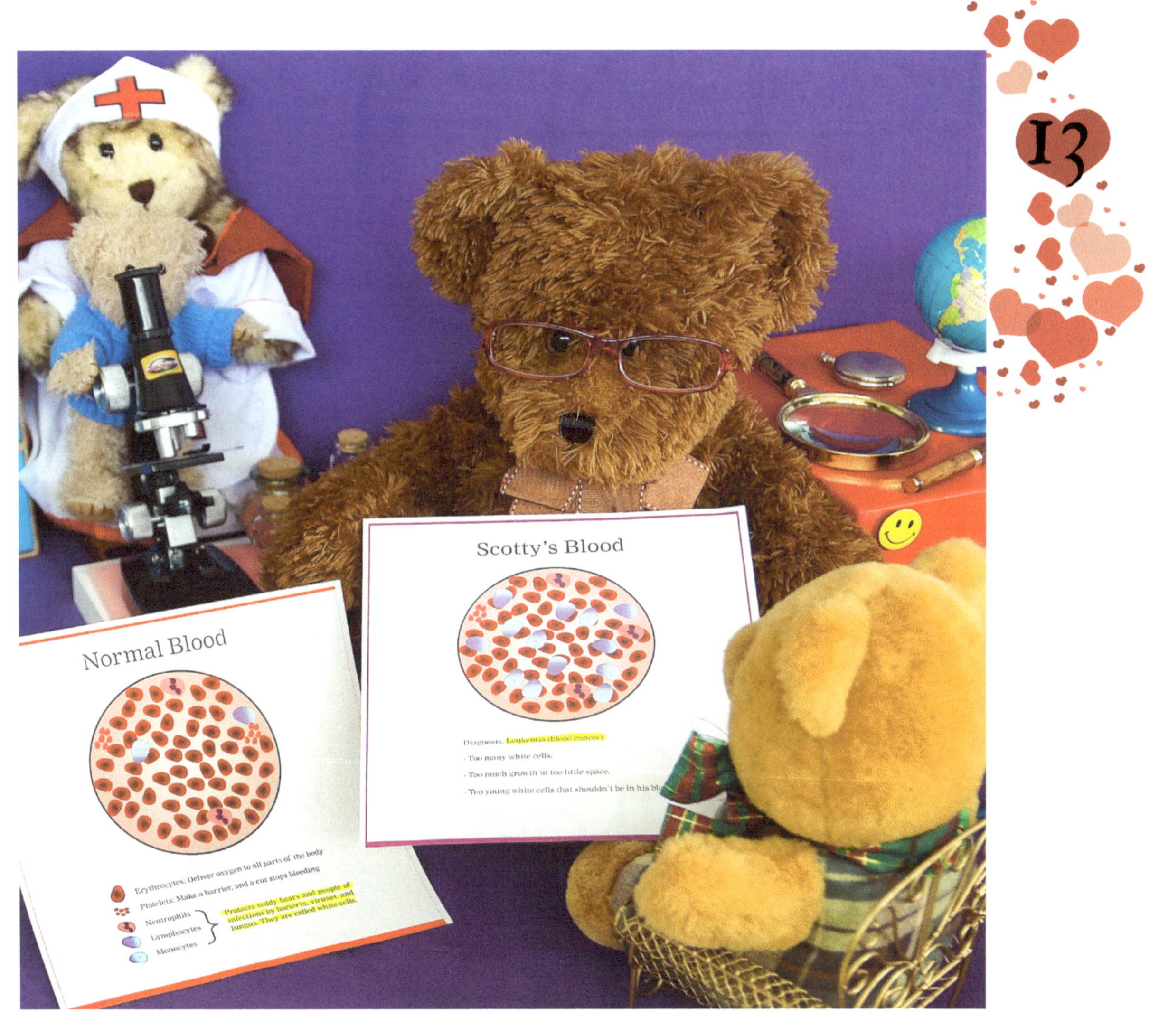

"They work to keep you healthy and multiply when necessary."

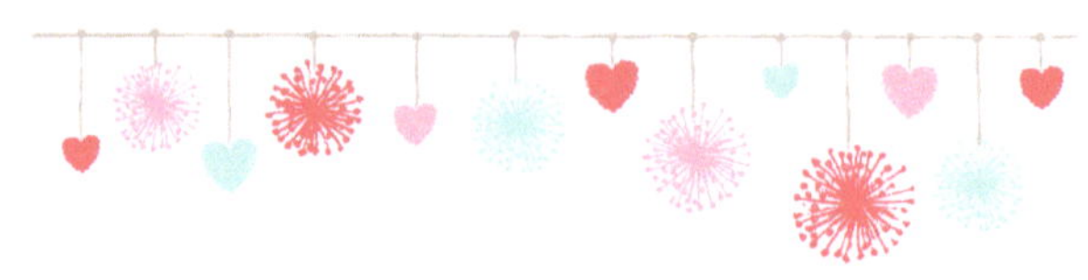

"Sometimes your cells stop working like they are supposed to, and begin multiplying and growing too fast. This is what we call cancer."

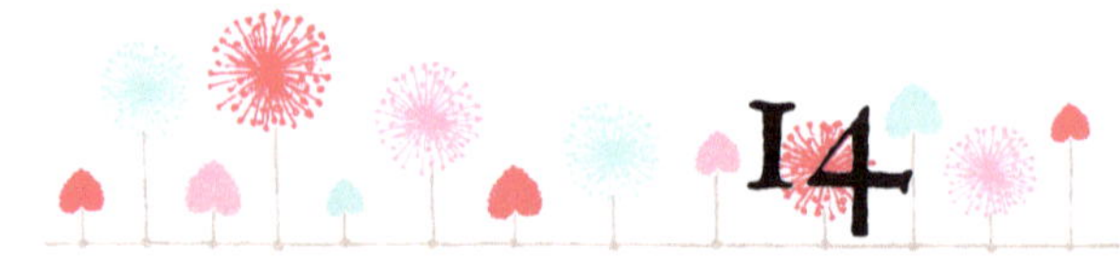

Normal Blood

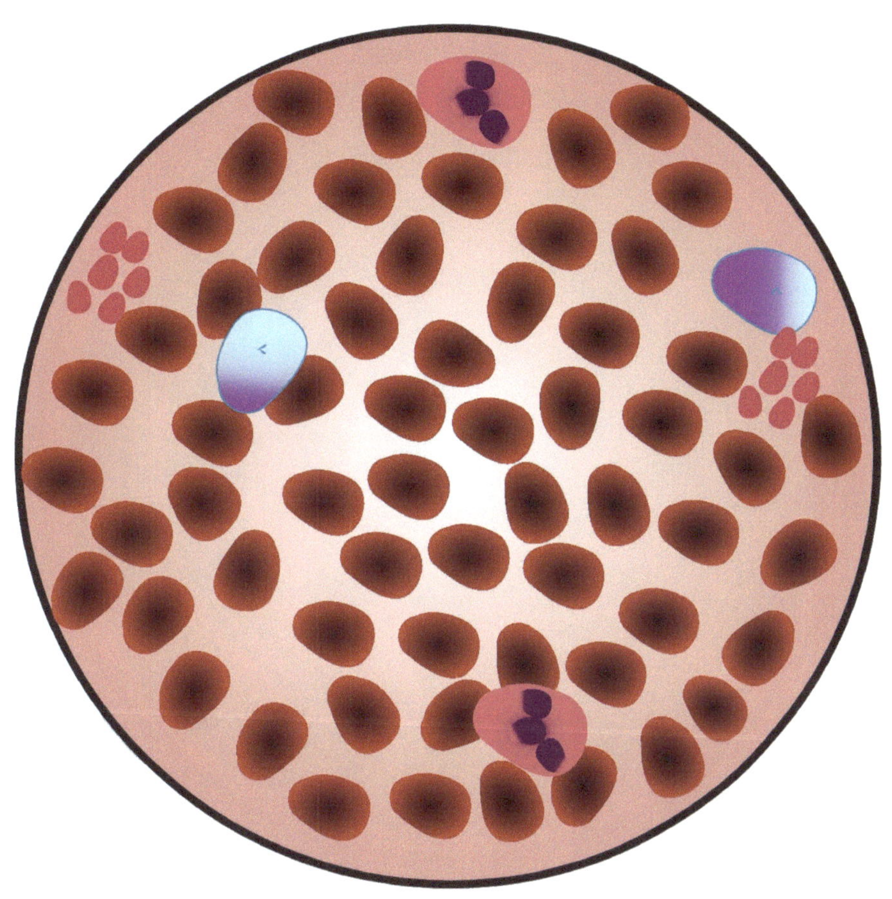

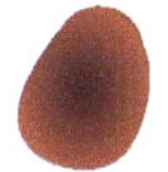 Erythrocytes: Deliver oxygen to all parts of the body

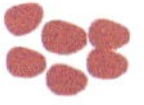 Platelets: Make a barrier, and a cut stops bleeding

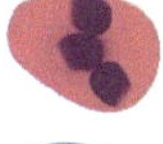 Neutrophils

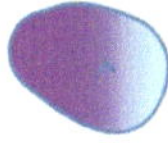 Lymphocytes

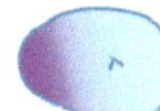 Monocytes

Protects teddy bears and people of infections by bacteria, viruses, and fungus. They are called white cells.

Scotty's Blood

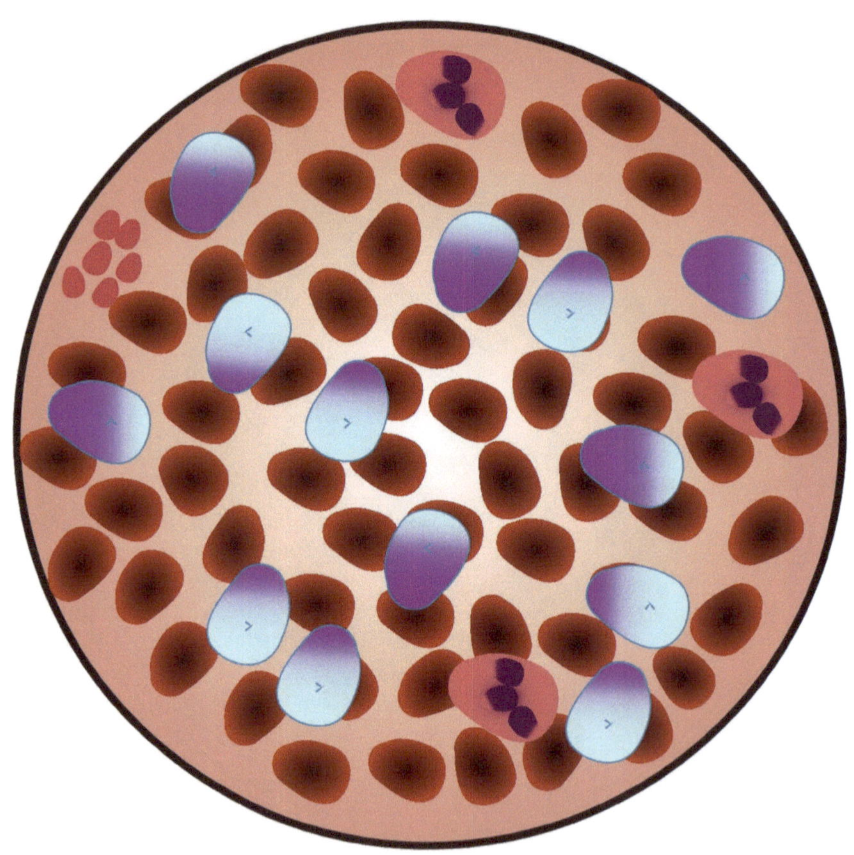

Diagnosis: Leukemia (blood cancer)

- Too many white cells.

- Too much growth in too little space.

- Too young white cells that shouldn´t be in his blood.

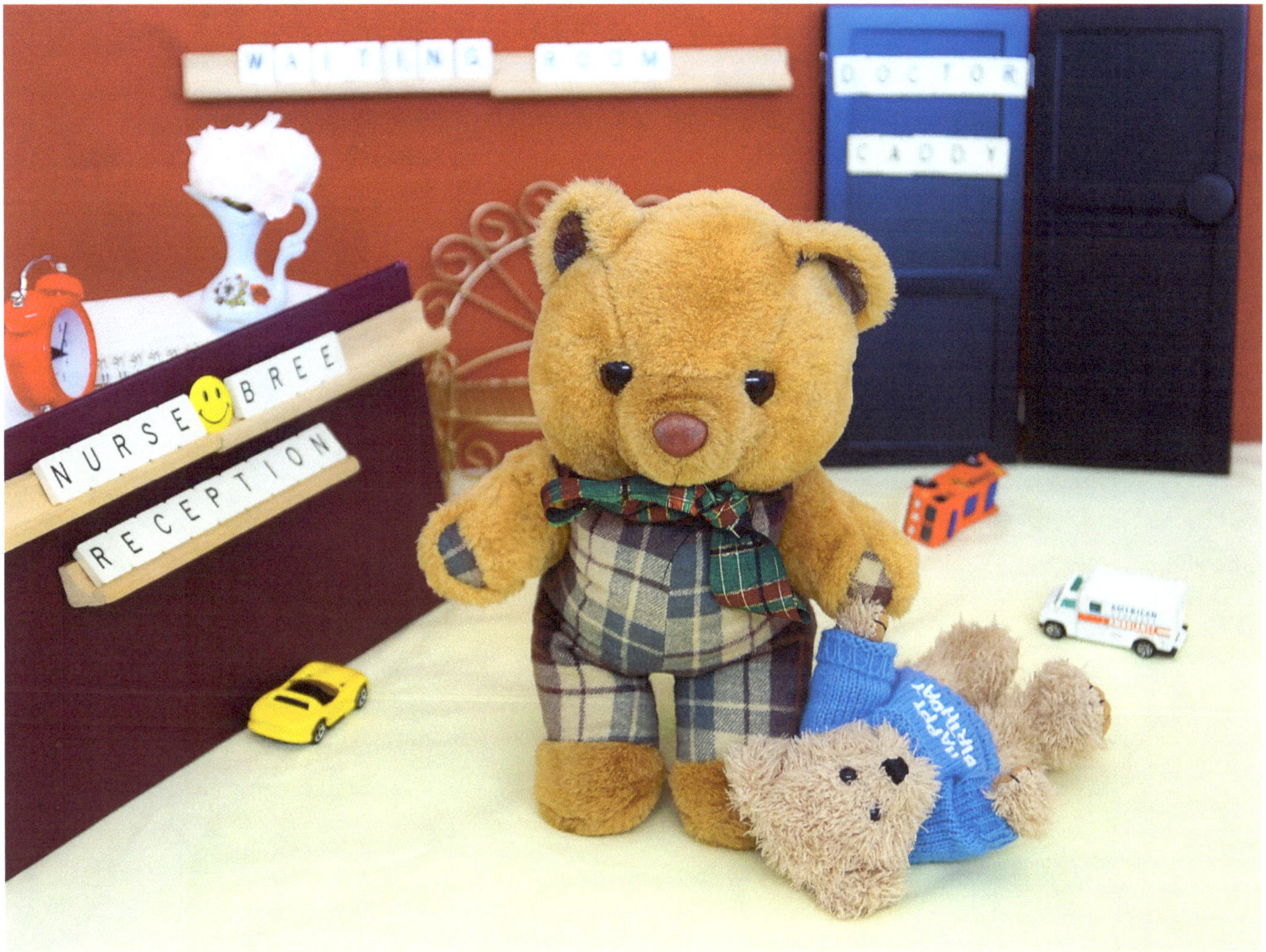

You feel alone...

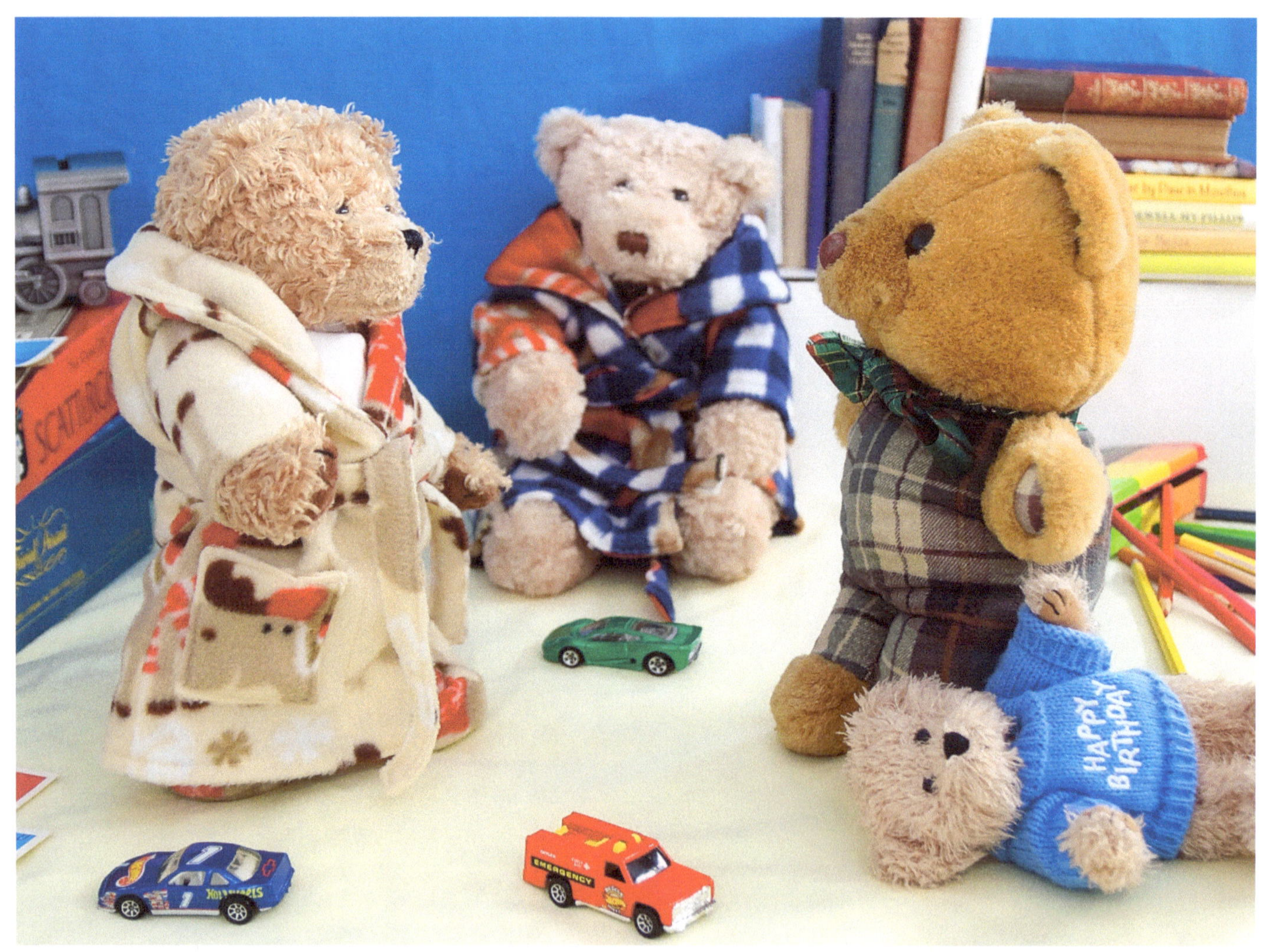

Until you realize that you are not
the only one.

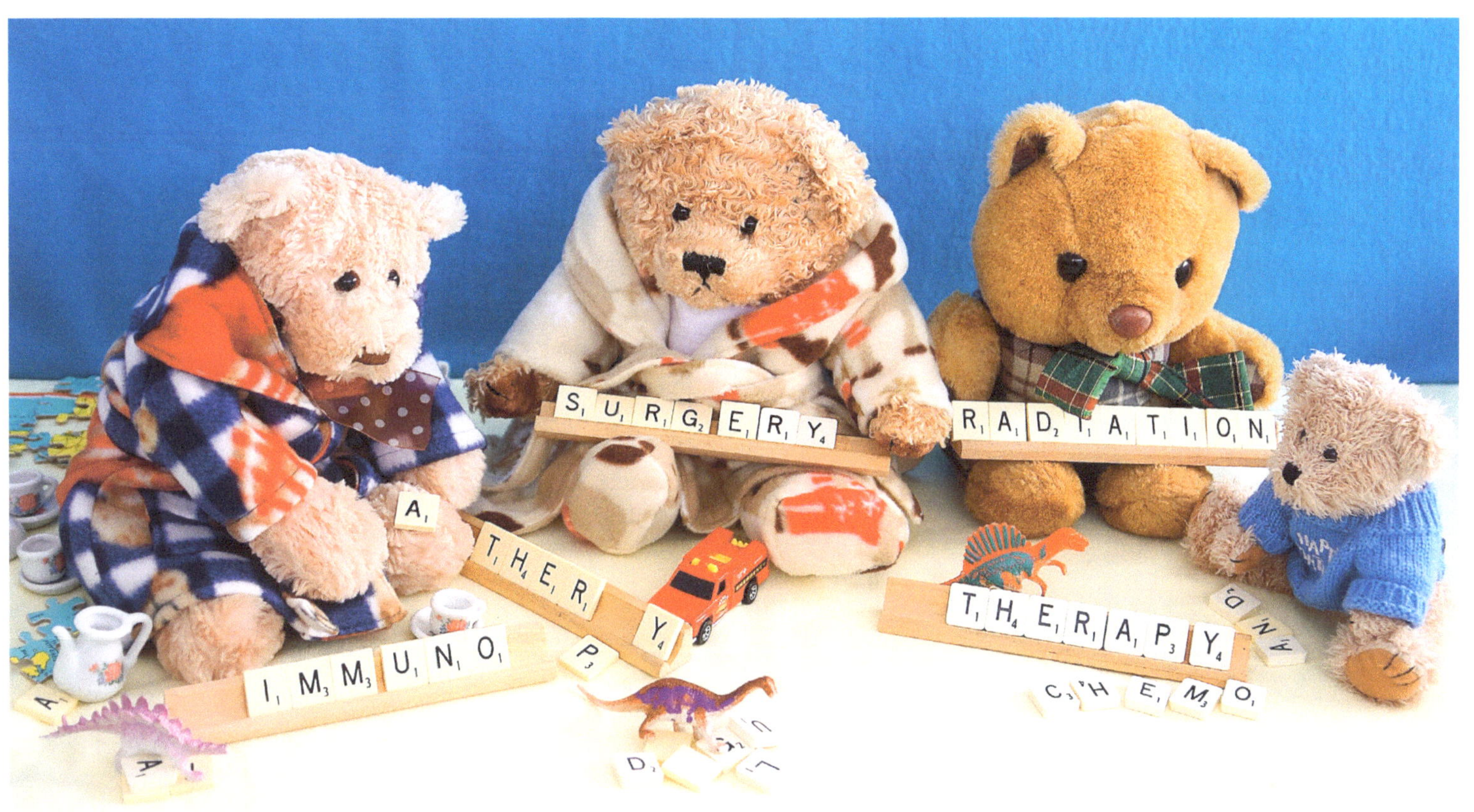

You can make new friends who are going through the same battle.

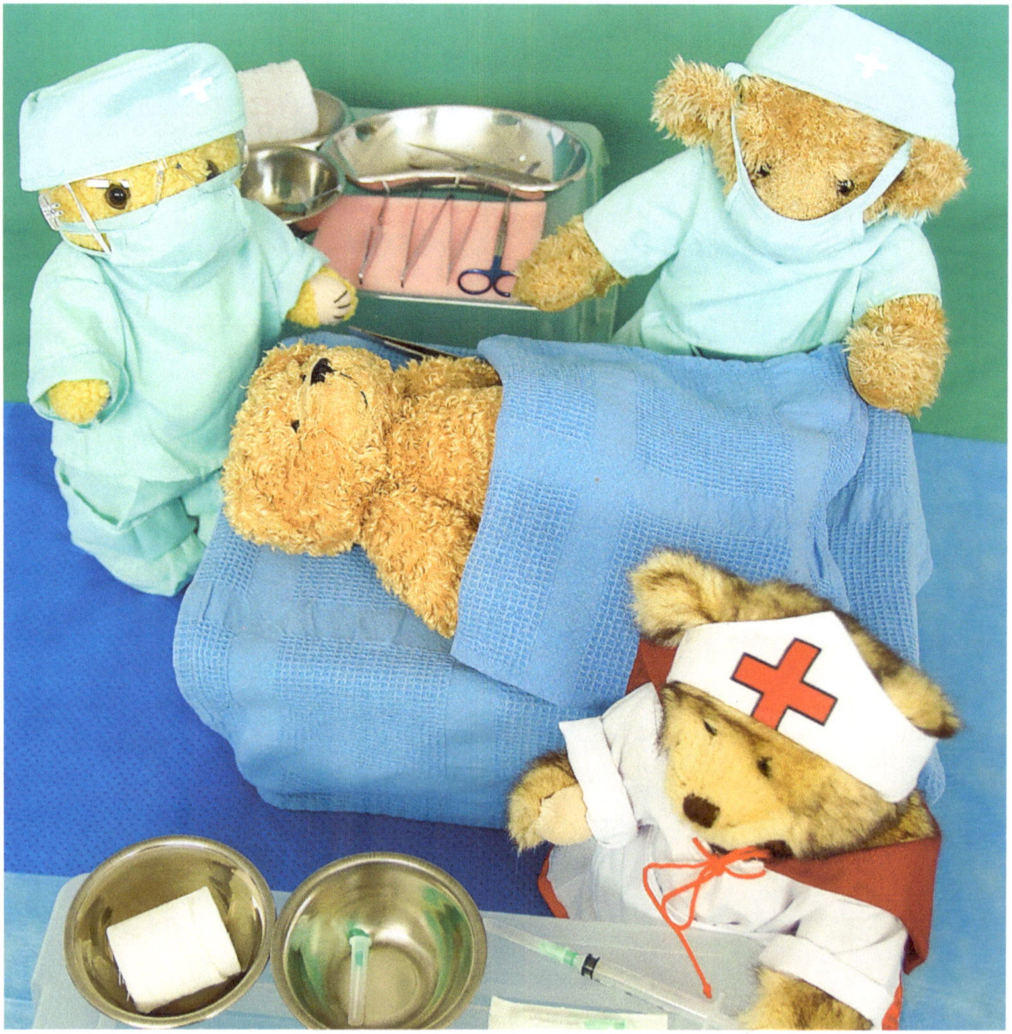

Some receive surgery to remove those crazy cells.

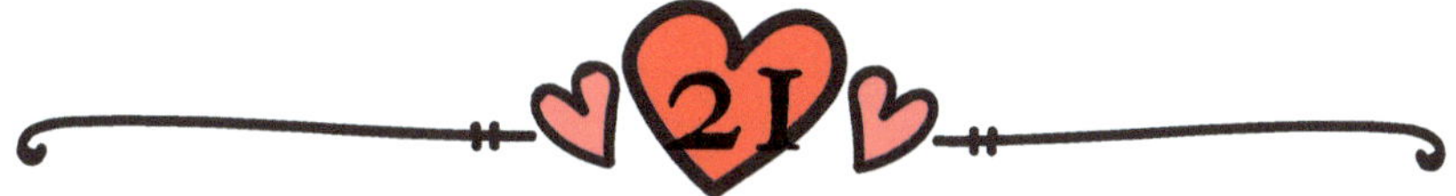

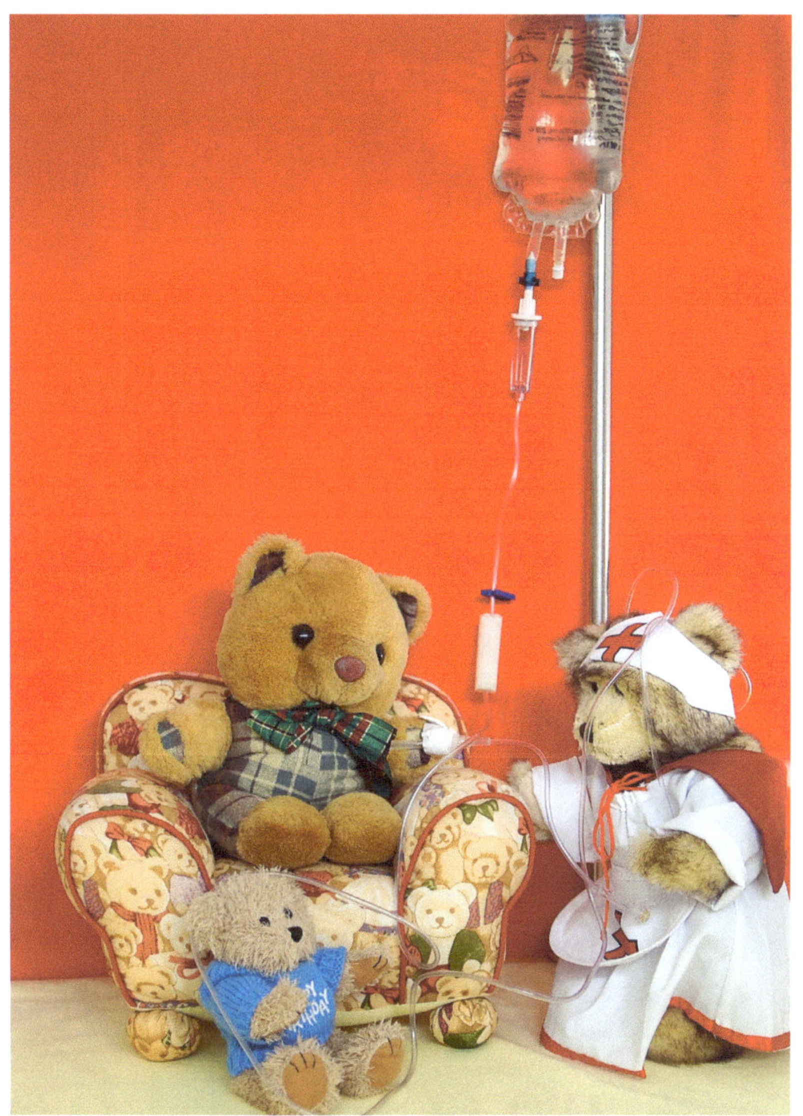

Others receive chemotherapy: a medicine to eliminate those crazy cells.

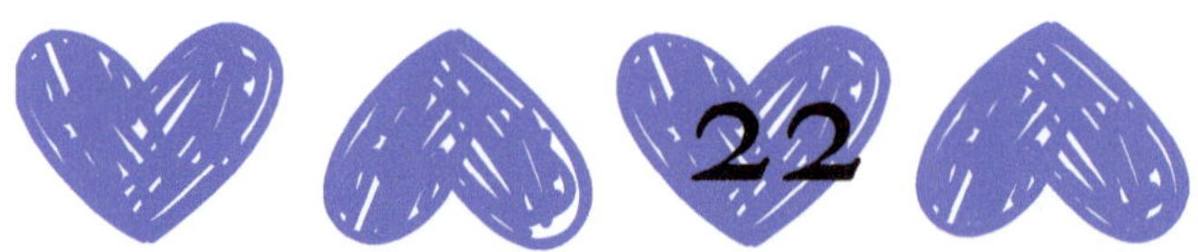

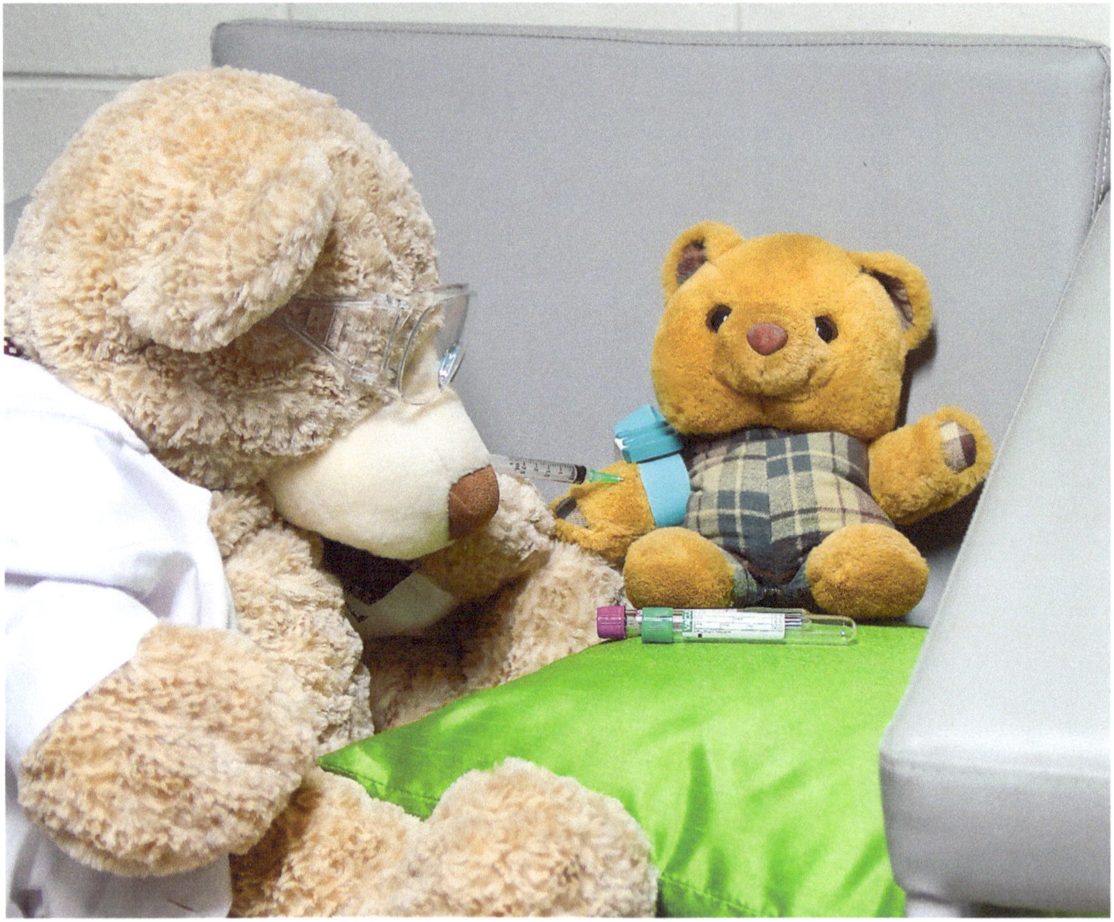

Some receive immunotherapy: good cells are collected from the blood through a tiny prick in the arm.

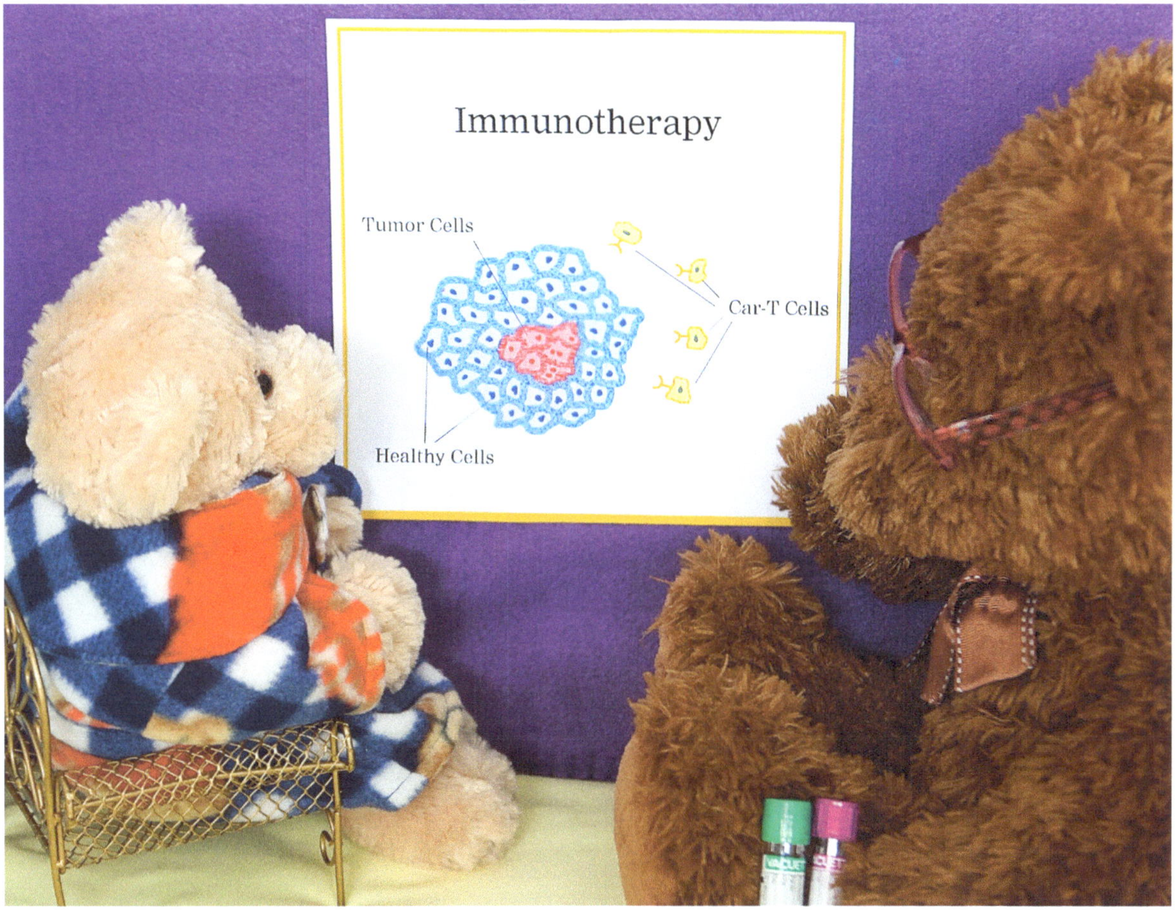

Then, they are changed in the laboratory to become super powerful cells. They will kill cells that don't work well.

Immunotherapy

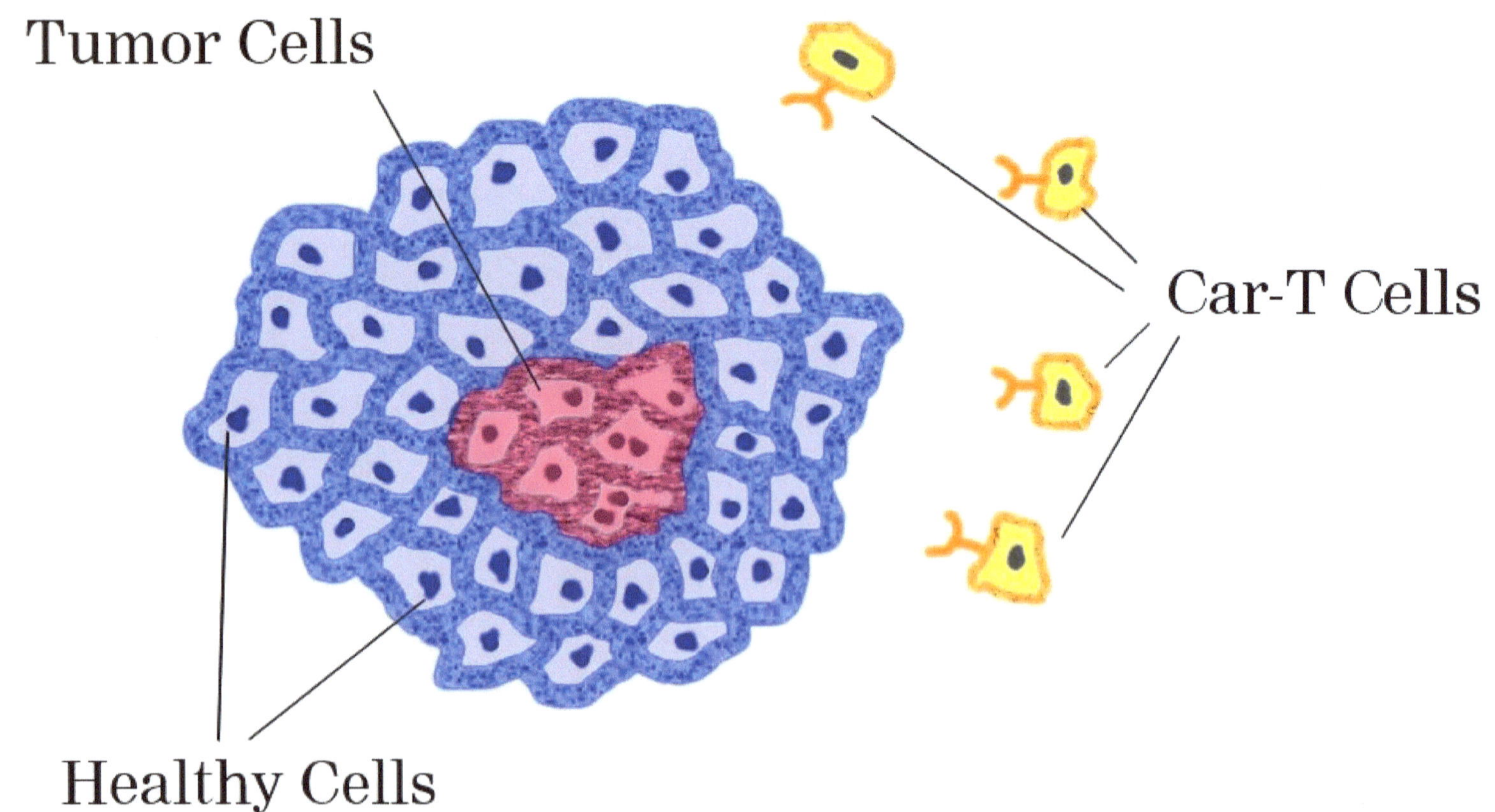

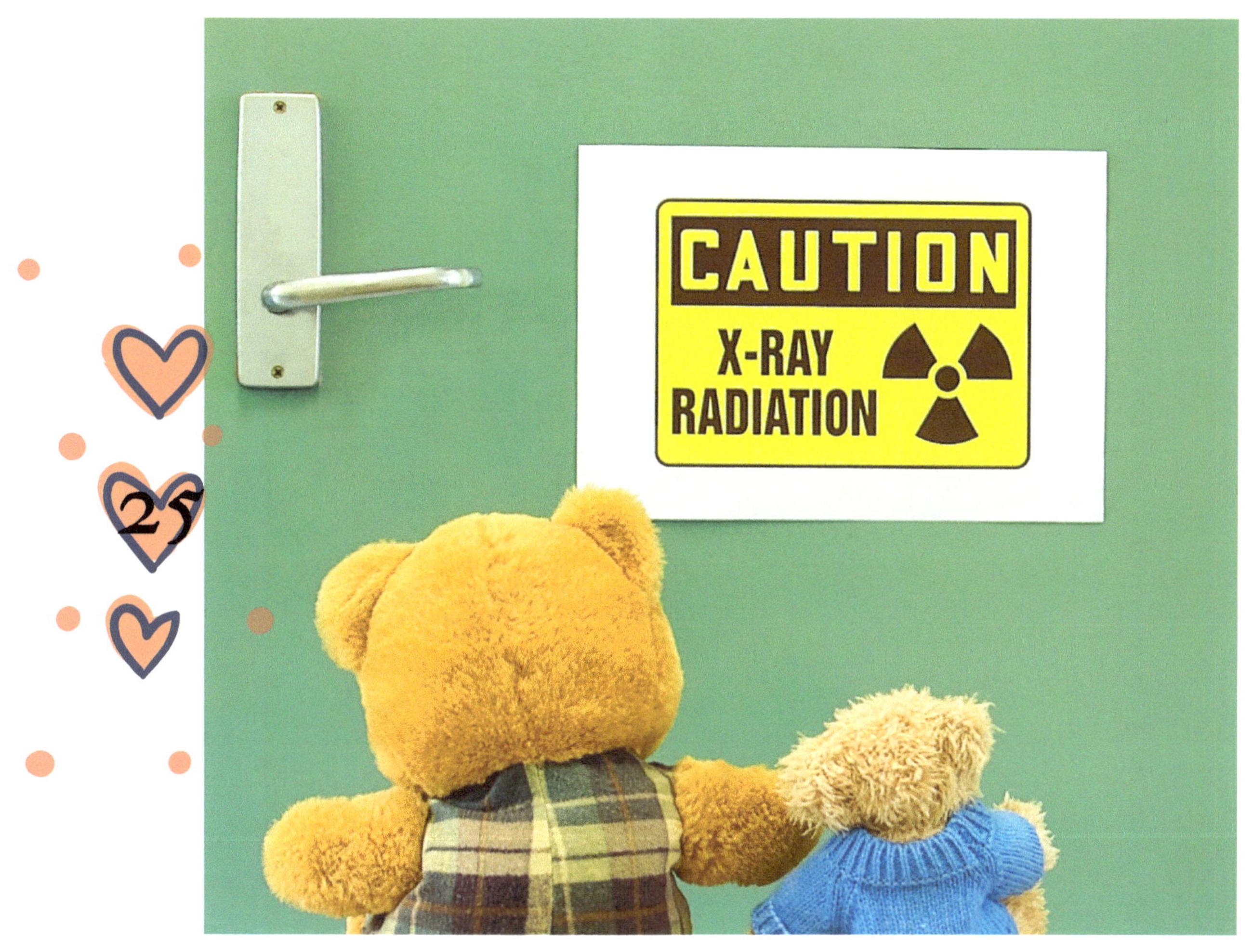

Others receive radiation: a super-powerful light that destroys cells that are not working well.

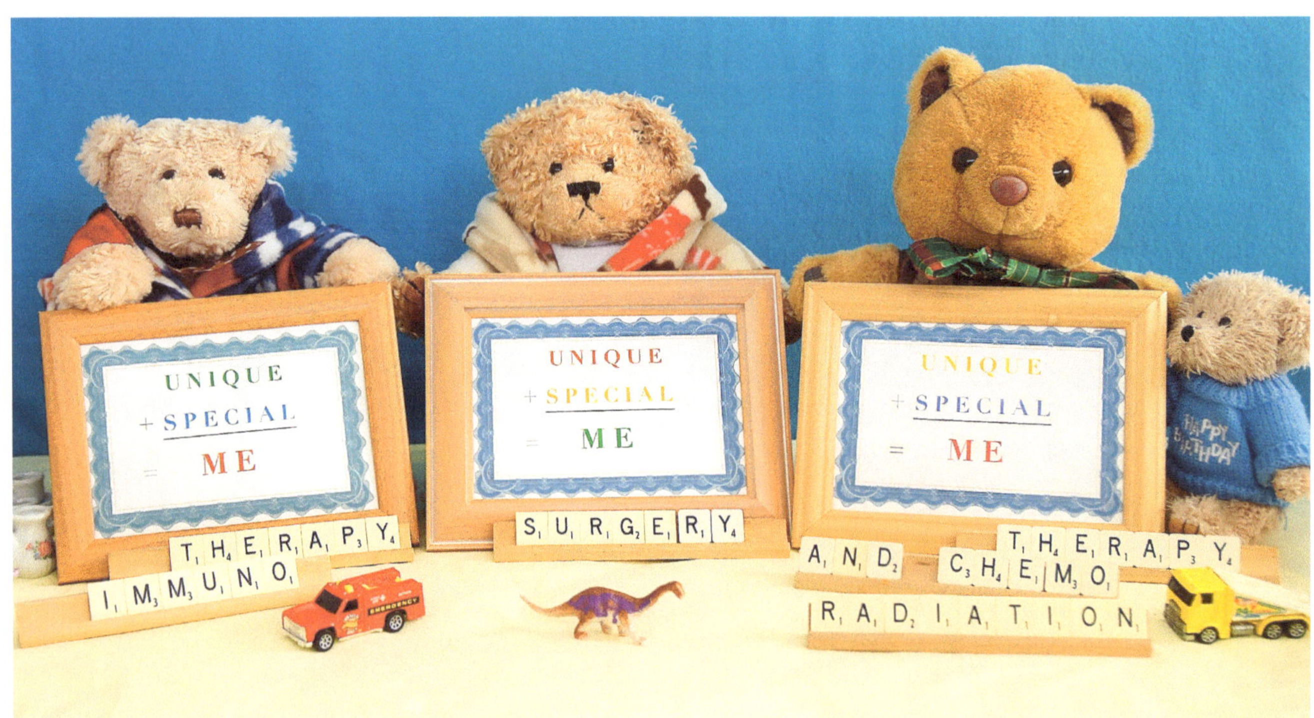

Everyone is unique and special. That's why the treatment is chosen specifically for each one.

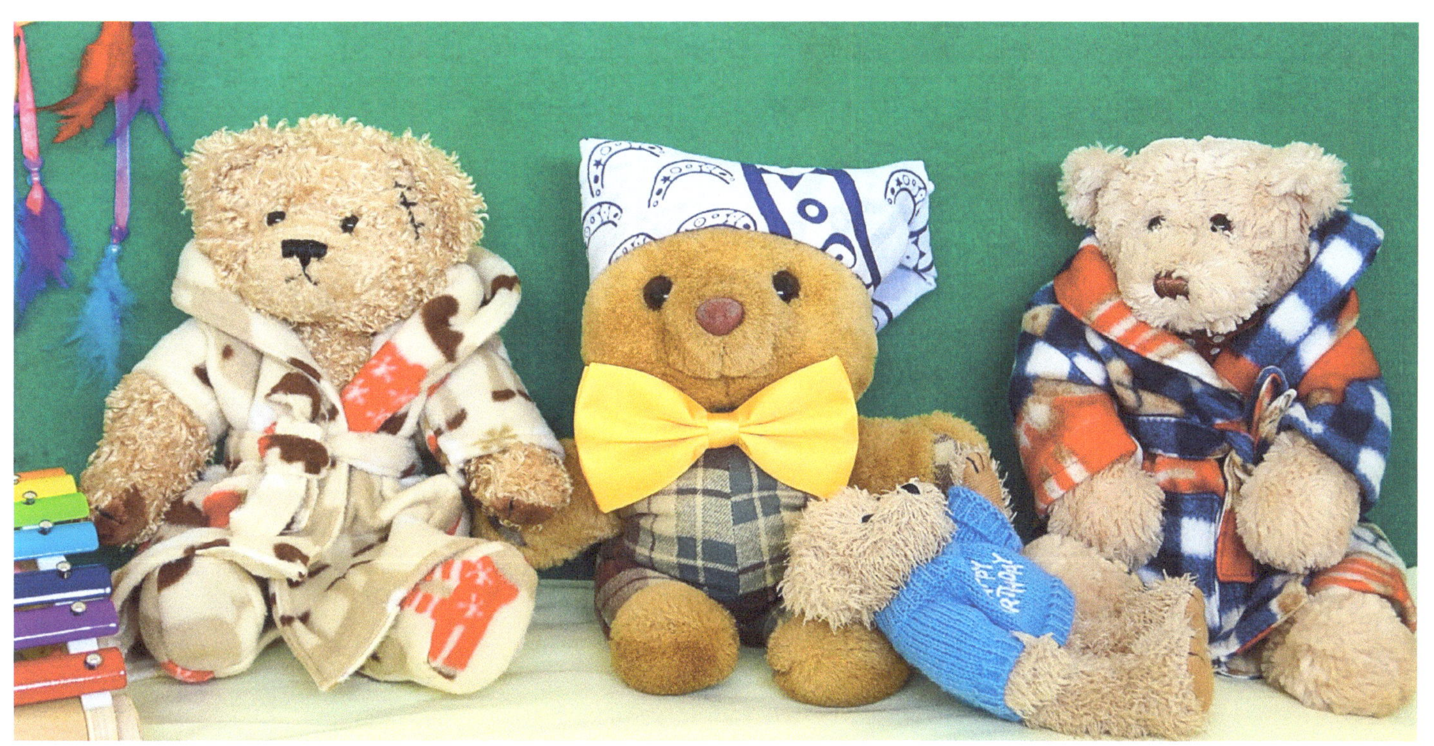

It's a special choice for a special bear.

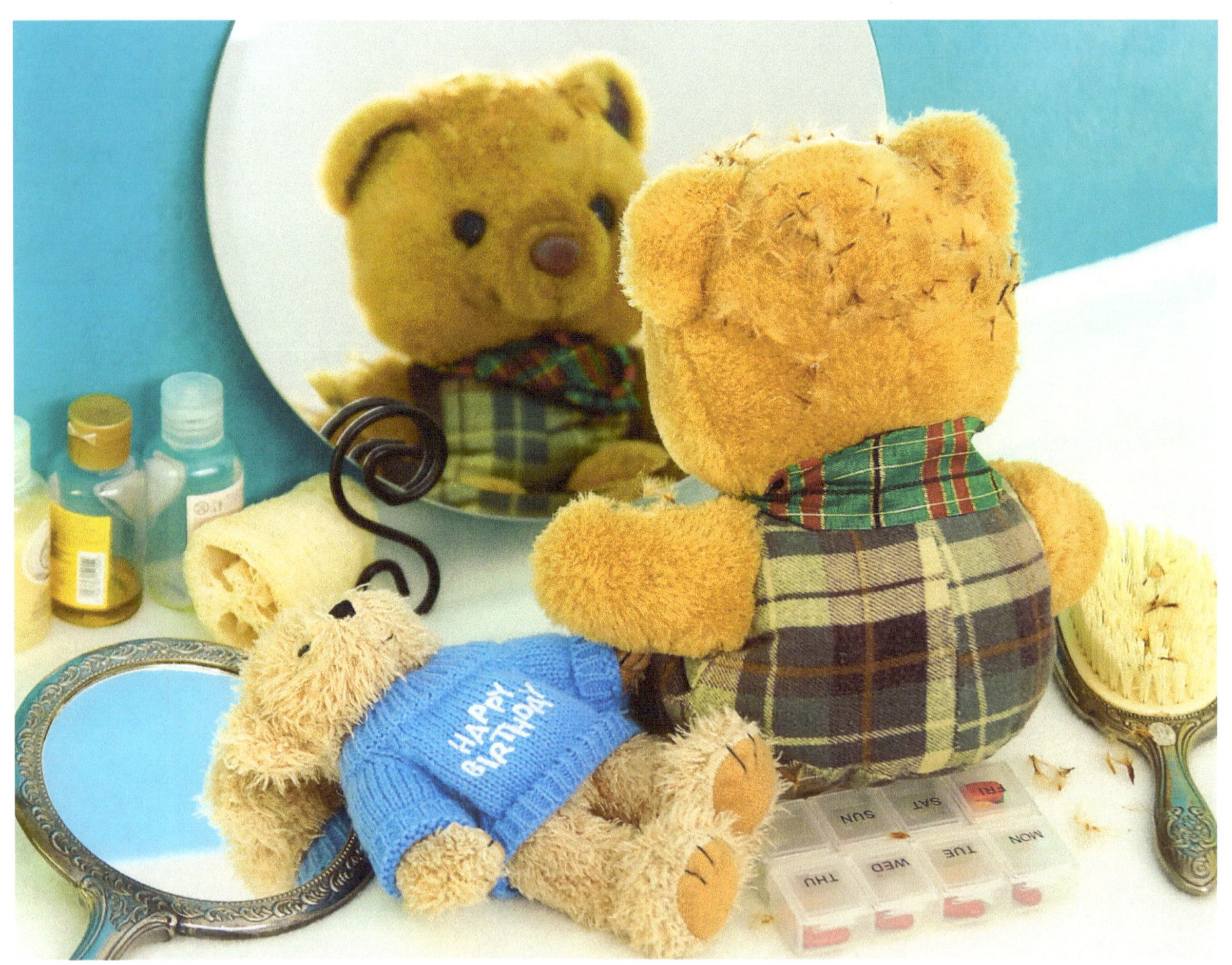

Sometimes, chemotherapy can cause hair loss because it is absorbed by the whole body during treatment.

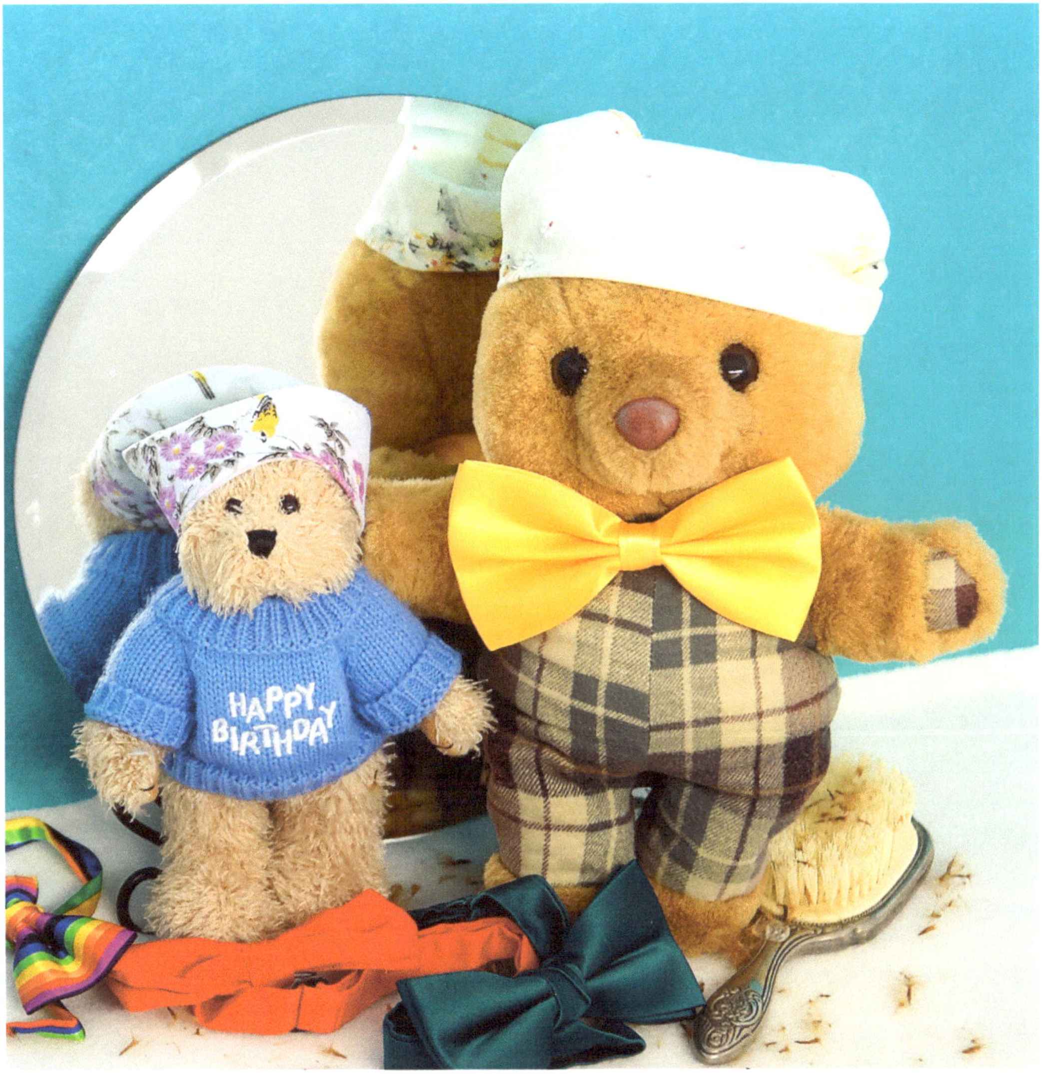

And sometimes radiation can cause hair loss, too.

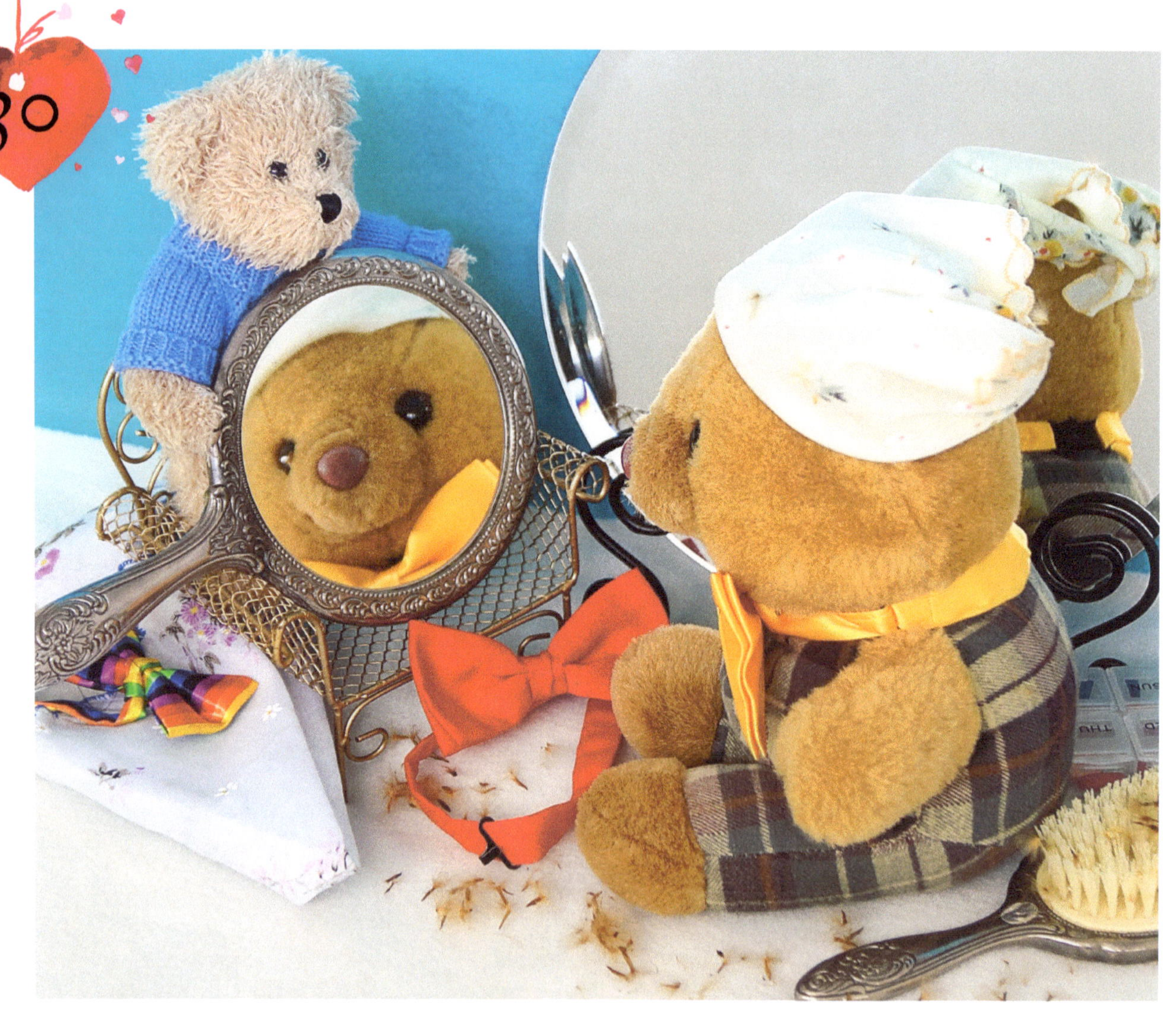

"My hair is gone. And I look different. But I still see ME."

31

"A wonderful, new, and beautiful me."

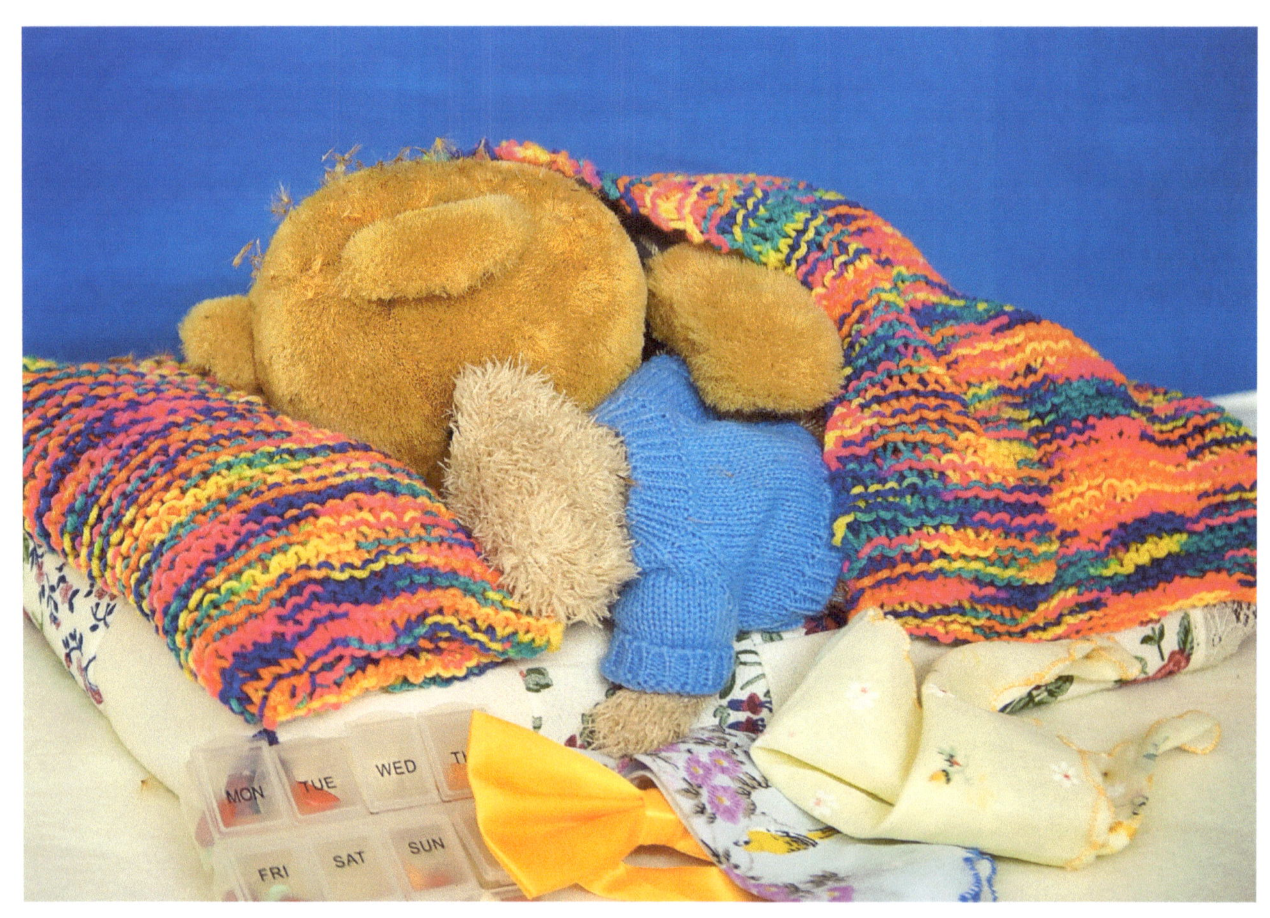

Sometimes, the treatment can be
exhausting.

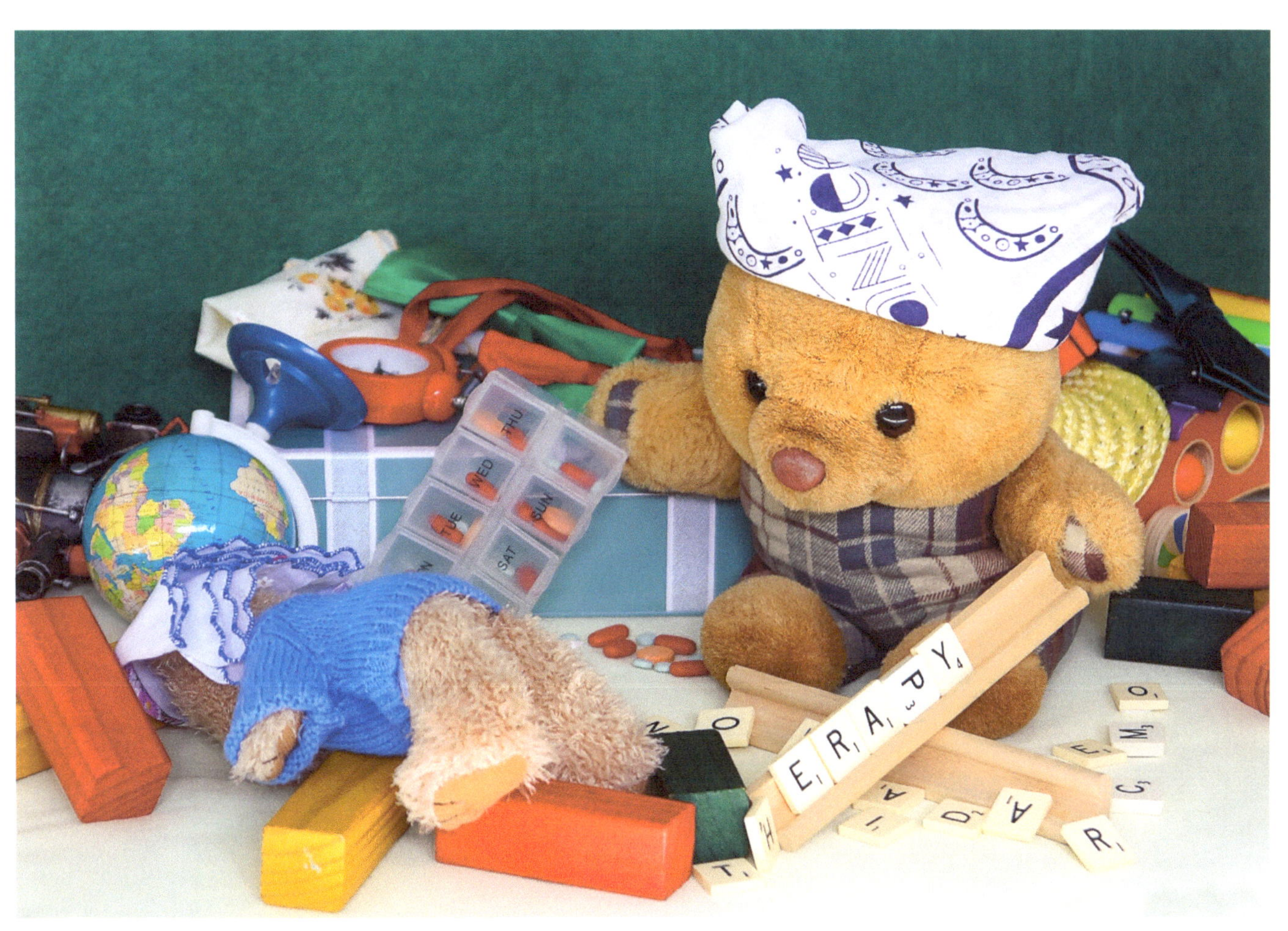

And maybe you'll be in a bad
mood.

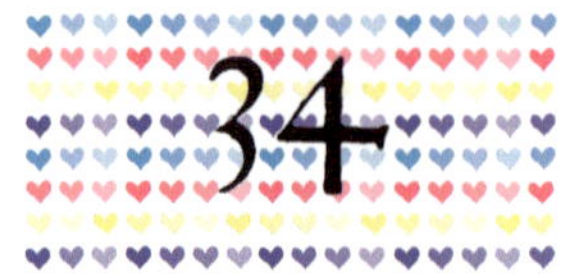

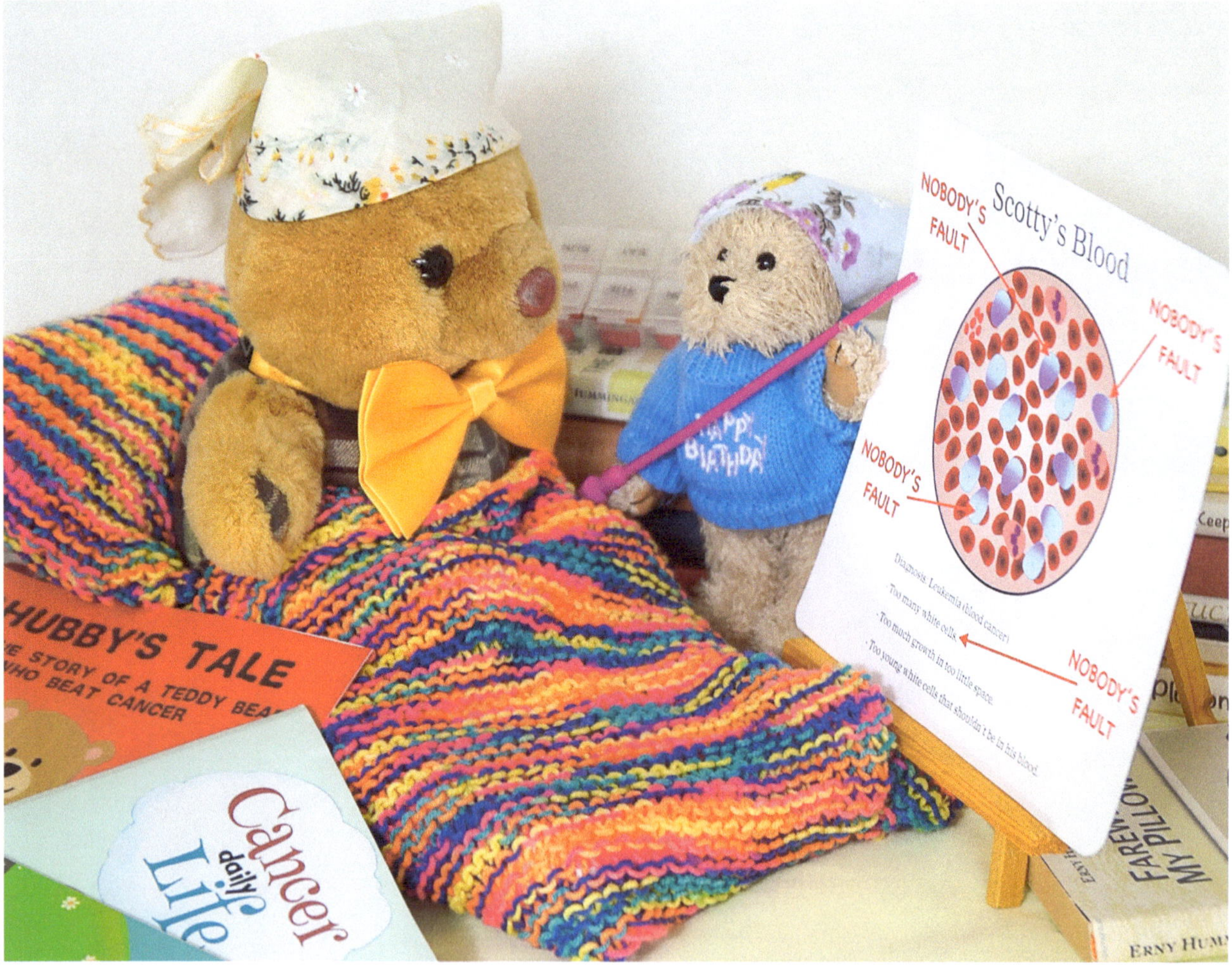

You should remember that it's nobody's fault...

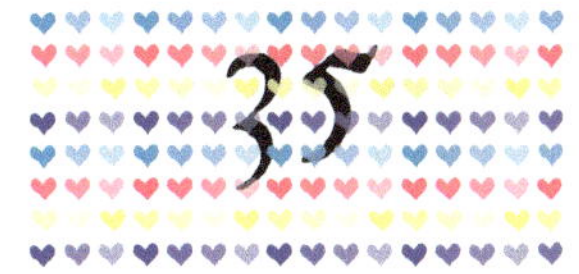

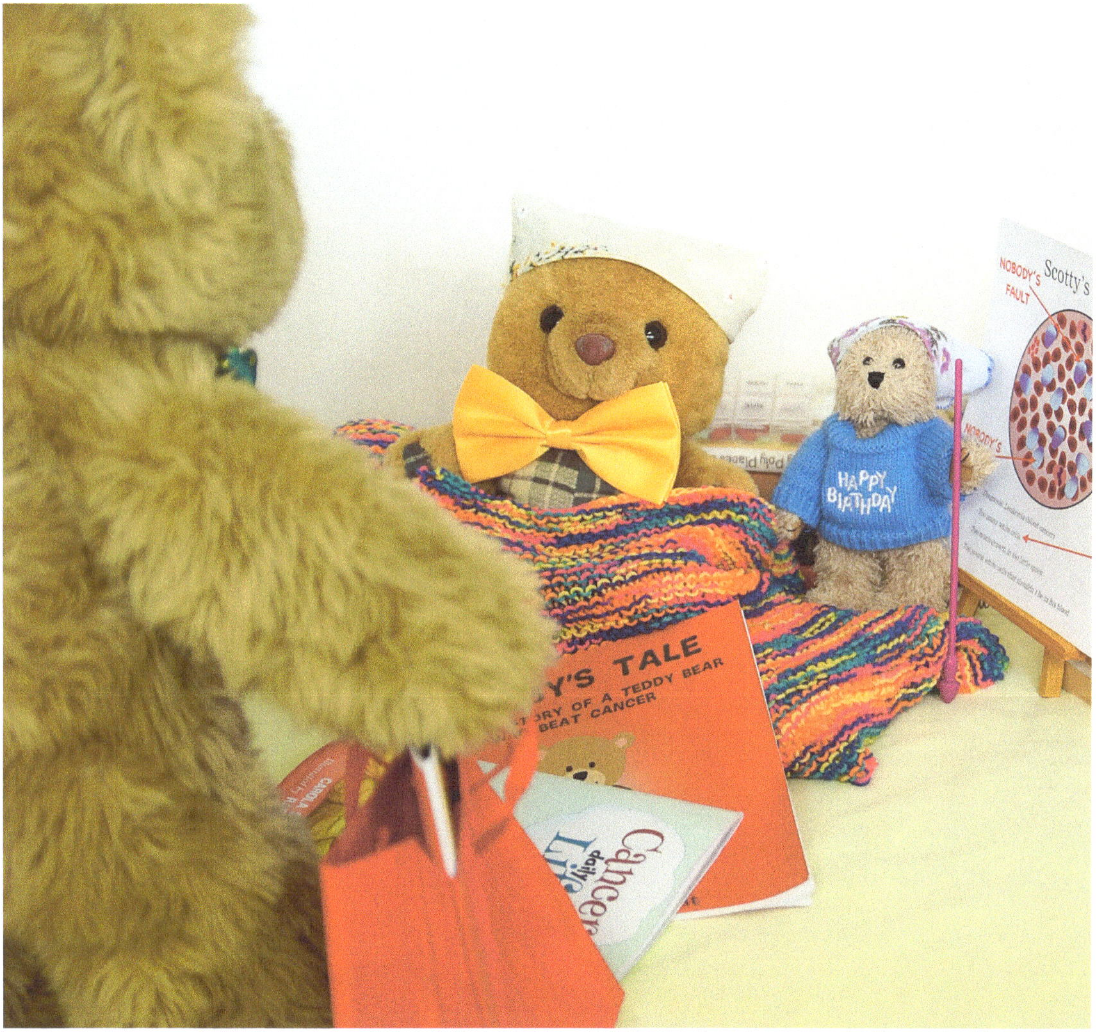

And the good moments will come
again soon.

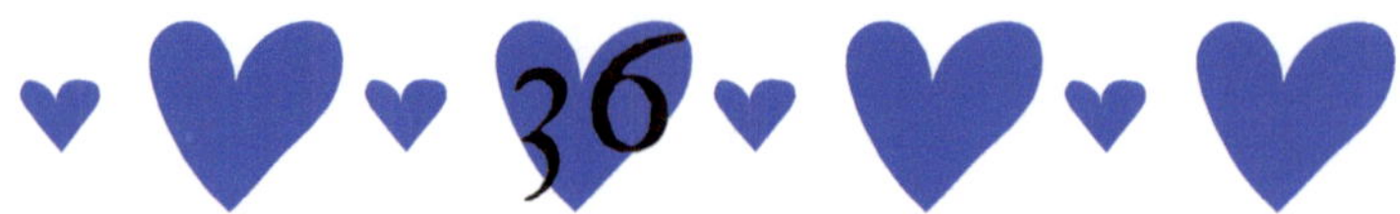

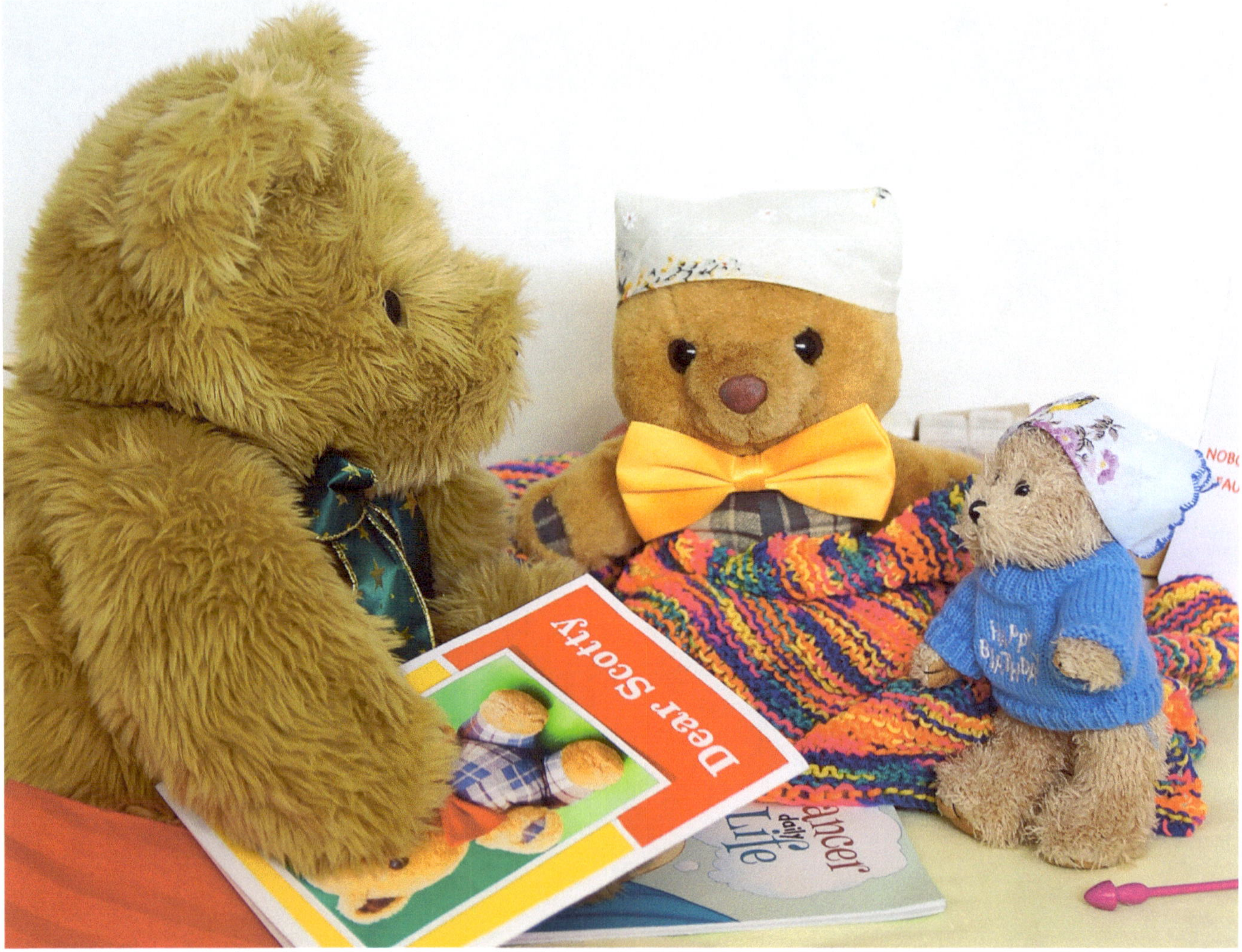

Maybe right now.

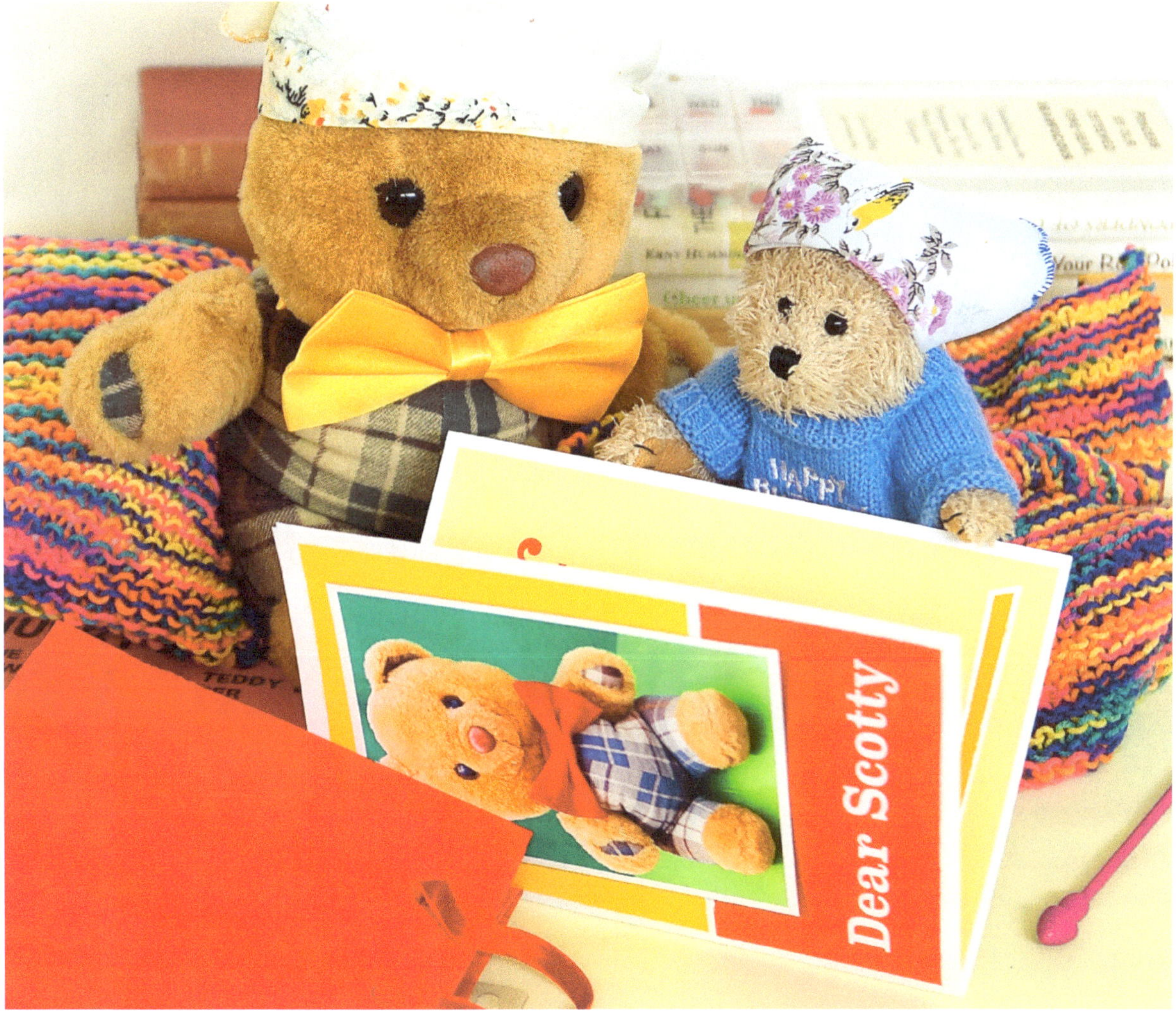

"Look, Scotty! A message for you!"

38

"Yay! What does it say, Little Teddy?"

"I don't know. I'm only your teddy bear. I don't know how to read!"

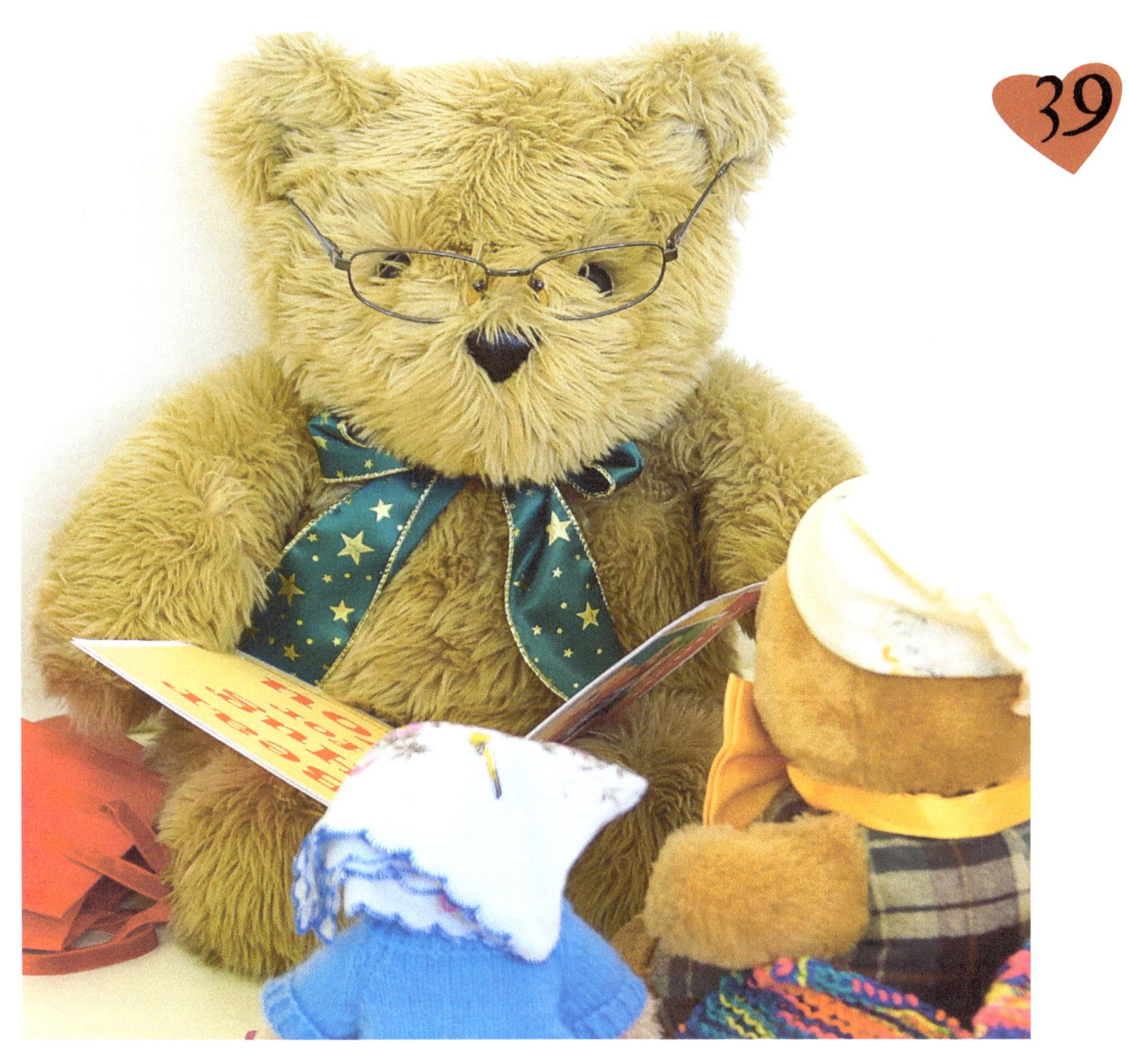

"I can read it for you, Scotty. Let me see…"

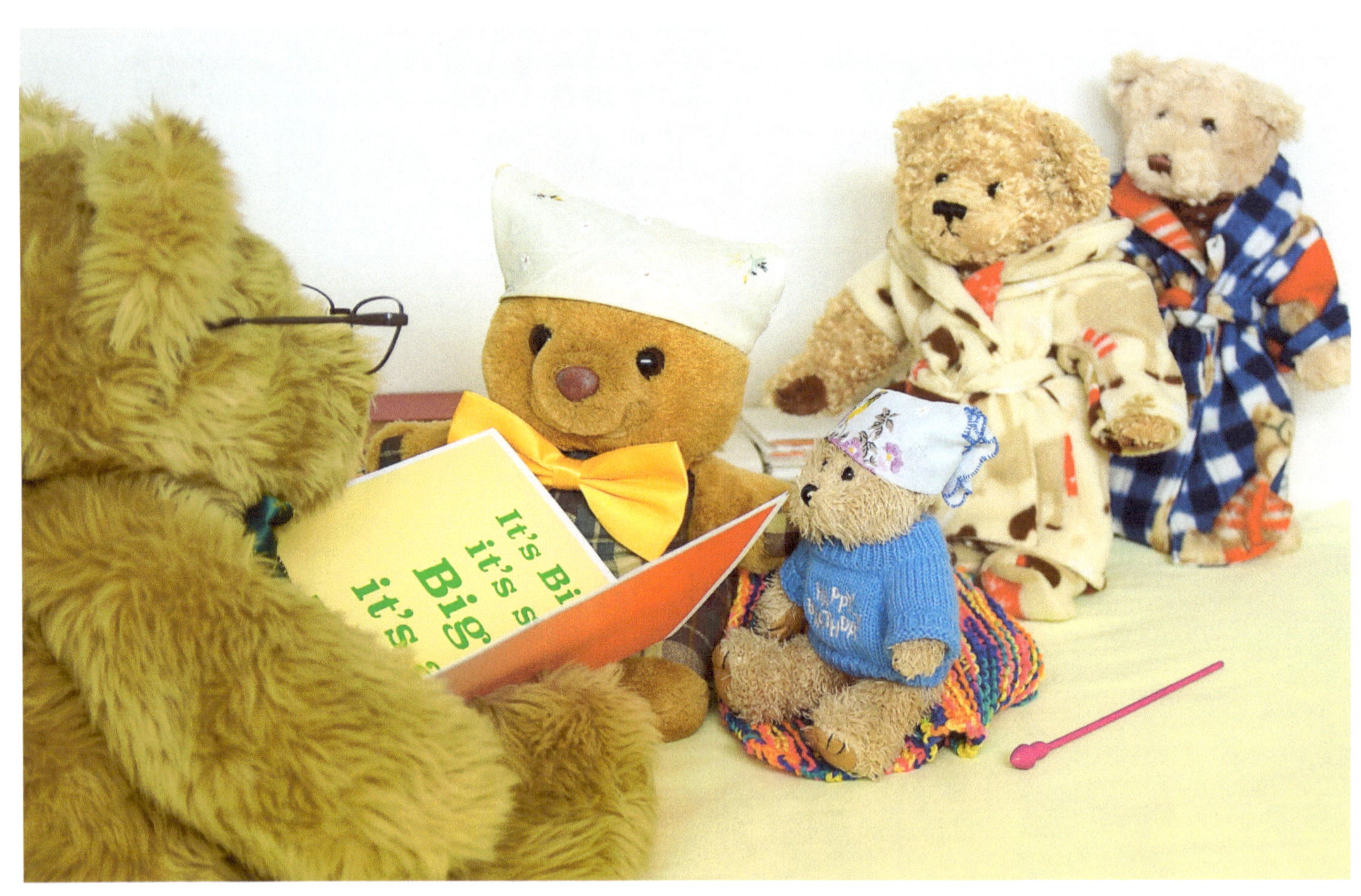

"It's a BIG..."

"A BIG what?"

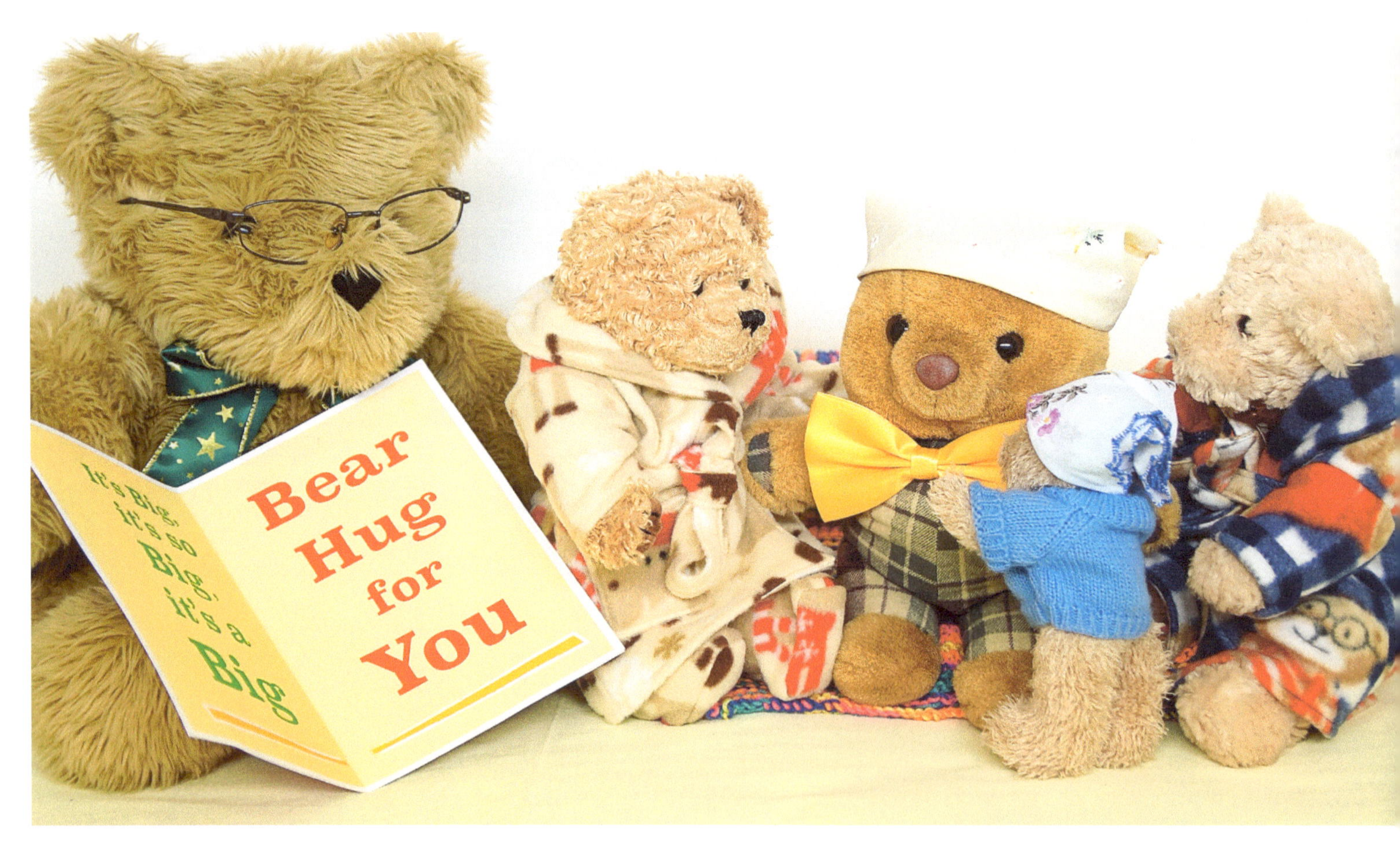

"A BIG BEAR HUG FOR YOU!"

9 798723 574601